Surgery: Complications, Risks and Consequences

Series Editor
Brendon J. Coventry

For further volumes:
http://www.springer.com/series/11761

Brendon J. Coventry

Editor

Lower Abdominal and Perineal Surgery

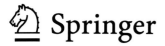 Springer

Editor
Brendon J. Coventry, BMBS, PhD,
FRACS, FACS, FRSM
Discipline of Surgery
Royal Adelaide Hospital
University of Adelaide
Adelaide, SA
Australia

ISBN 978-1-4471-5468-6   ISBN 978-1-4471-5469-3   (eBook)
DOI 10.1007/978-1-4471-5469-3
Springer London Heidelberg New York Dordrecht

Library of Congress Control Number: 2013957696

Printed on acid-free paper

Springer is part of Springer Science+Business Media (www.springer.com)

*This book is dedicated to my wonderful wife
Christine and children Charles, Cameron,
Alexander and Eloise who make me so
proud, having supported me through this
mammoth project; my patients, past, present
and future; my numerous mentors, teachers,
colleagues, friends and students, who know
who they are; my parents Beryl and
Lawrence; and my parents-in-law Barbara
and George, all of whom have taught me and
encouraged me to achieve*

*"Without love and understanding we have
but nothing"*

Brendon J. Coventry

Foreword I

This comprehensive treatise is remarkable for its breadth and scope and its authorship by global experts. Indeed, knowledge of its content is essential if we are to achieve optimal and safe outcomes for our patients. The content embodies the details of our surgical discipline and how to incorporate facts and evidence into our surgical judgment as well as recommendations to our patients.

While acknowledging that the technical aspects of surgery are its distinguishing framework of our profession, the art and judgment of surgery requires an in depth knowledge of biology, anatomy, pathophysiology, clinical science, surgical outcomes and complications that distinguishes the theme of this book. This knowledge is essential to assure us that we are we doing the right operation, at the right time, and in the right patient. In turn, that knowledge is essential to take into account how surgical treatment interfaces with the correct sequence and combination with other treatment modalities. It is also essential to assess the extent of scientific evidence from clinical trials and surgical expertise that is the underpinning of our final treatment recommendation to our patient.

Each time I sit across from a patient to make a recommendation for a surgical treatment, I am basing my recommendation on a "benefit/risk ratio" that integrates scientific evidence, and my intuition gained through experience. That is, do the potential benefits outweigh the potential risks and complications as applied to an individual patient setting? The elements of that benefit/ risk ratio that are taken into account include: the natural history of the disease, the stage/extent of disease, scientific and empirical evidence of treatment outcomes, quality of life issues (as perceived by the patient), co-morbidity that might influence surgical outcome, risks and complications inherent to the operation (errors of commission) and the risk(s) of not proceeding with an operation (errors of omission).

Thus, if we truly want to improve our surgical outcomes, then we must understand and be able to either avoid, or execute sound management of, any complications that occur (regardless of whether they are due to co-morbidity or iatrogenic causes), to get our patent safely through the operation and its post-operative course. These subjects are nicely incorporated into the content of this book.

I highly recommend this book as a practical yet comprehensive treatise for the practicing surgeon and the surgical trainee. It is well organized, written with great clarity and nicely referenced when circumstances require further information.

Charles M. Balch, MD, FACS
Professor of Surgery
University of Texas, Southwestern Medical Center,
Dallas, TX, USA
Formerly, Professor of Surgery, Johns Hopkins Hospital,
Baltimore, MD, USA
Formerly, Executive Vice President and CEO,
American Society of Clinical Oncology (ASCO)
Past-President, Society of Surgical Oncology (USA)

Foreword II

Throughout my clinical academic career I have aspired to improve the quality and safety of my surgical and clinical practice. It is very clear, while reading this impressive collection and synthesis of high-impact clinical evidence and international expert consensus, that in this new textbook, Brendon Coventry has the ambition to innovate and advance the quality and safety of surgical discipline.

In these modern times, where we find an abundance of information that is available through the internet, and of often doubtful authenticity, it is vital that we retain a professional responsibility for the collection, analysis and dissemination of evidenced-based and accurate knowledge and guidance to benefit both clinicians and our patients.

This practical and broad-scoped compendium, which contains over 250 procedures and their related complications and associated risks, will undoubtedly become a benchmark to raise the safety and quality of surgical practice for all that read it. It also manages to succeed in providing a portal for all surgeons, at any stage of their careers, to reflect on the authors' own combined experiences and the collective insights of a strong and influential network of peers.

This text emphasizes the need to understand and appreciate our patients and the intimate relationship that their physiology, co-morbidities and underlying diagnosis can have upon their unique surgical risk with special regard to complications and adverse events.

I recognize that universally across clinical practice and our profession, the evidence base and guidance to justify our decision-making is growing, but there is also a widening gap between what we know and what we do. The variation that we see in the quality of practice throughout the world should not be tolerated.

This text makes an assertive contribution to promote quality by outlining the prerequisite foundational knowledge of surgery, science and anatomy and their complex interactions with clinical outcome that is needed for all in the field of surgery.

I thoroughly recommend this expertly constructed collection. Its breadth and quality is a testament to its authors and editor.

Professor the Lord Ara Darzi, PC, KBE, FRCS, FRS
Paul Hamlyn Chair of Surgery
Imperial College London, London, UK
Formerly Undersecretary of State for Health,
Her Majesty's Government, UK

Conditions of Use and Disclaimer

Information is provided *for improved medical education and potential improvement in clinical practice only.* The information is based on composite material from research studies and professional personal opinion and does not guarantee accuracy for any specific clinical situation or procedure. There is also *no express or implied guarantee to accuracy or that surgical complications will be prevented, minimized, or reduced* in any way. The advice is *intended for use by individuals with suitable professional qualifications* and education in medical practice and the ability to apply the knowledge in a suitable manner for a specific condition or disease, and in an appropriate clinical context. The data is complex by nature and open to some interpretation. The purpose is to assist medical practitioners to improve awareness of possible complications, risks or consequences associated with surgical procedures for the benefit of those practitioners in the improved care of their patients. The application of the information contained herein for a specific patient or problem must be performed with care to ensure that the situation and advice is appropriate and correct for that patient and situation. The material is expressly *not for medicolegal purposes.*

The information contained in *Surgery: Complications, Risks and Consequences* is provided for the purpose of improving consent processes in healthcare and in no way guarantees prevention, early detection, risk reduction, economic benefit or improved practice of surgical treatment of any disease or condition.

The information provided in *Surgery: Complications, Risks and Consequences* is of a general nature and is not a substitute for independent medical advice or research in the management of particular diseases or patient situations by health care professionals. It should not be taken as replacing or overriding medical advice.

The Publisher or *Copyright* holder does not accept any liability for any injury, loss, delay or damage incurred arising from use, misuse, interpretation, omissions or reliance on the information provided in *Surgery: Complications, Risks and Consequences* directly or indirectly.

Currency and Accuracy of Information

The user should always check that any information acted upon is up-to-date and accurate. Information is provided in good faith and is **subject to change and alteration without notice**. Every effort is made with *Surgery: Complications, Risks and Consequences* to provide current information, but no warranty, guarantee or legal responsibility is given that information provided or referred to has not changed without the knowledge of the publisher, editor or authors. Always check the quality of information provided or referred to for accuracy for the situation where it is intended to be used, or applied. We do, however, attempt to provide useful and valid information. Because of the broad nature of the information provided incompleteness or omissions of specific or general complications may have occured and users must take this into account when using the text. No responsibility is taken for delayed, missed or inaccurate diagnosis of any illness, disease or health state at any time.

External Web Site Links or References

The decisions about the accuracy, currency, reliability and correctness of information made by individuals using the *Surgery: Complications, Risks and Consequences* information or from external Internet links remain the individuals own concern and responsibility. Such external links or reference materials or other information should not be taken as an endorsement, agreement or recommendation of any third party products, services, material, information, views or content offered by these sites or publications. Users should check the sources and validity of information obtained for themselves prior to use.

Privacy and Confidentiality

We maintain confidentiality and privacy of personal information but do not guarantee any confidentiality or privacy.

Errors or Suggested Changes

If you or any colleagues note any errors or wish to suggest changes please notify us directly as they would be gratefully received.

How to Use This Book

This book provides a resource for better understanding of surgical procedures and potential complications in general terms. The application of this material will depend on the individual patient and clinical context. It is not intended to be absolutely comprehensive for all situations or for all patients, but act as a 'guide' for understanding and prediction of complications, to assist in risk management and improvement of patient outcomes.

The design of the book is aimed at:

- Reducing Risk and better Managing Risks associated with surgery
- Providing information about 'general complications' associated with surgery
- Providing information about 'specific complications' associated with surgery
- Providing comprehensive information in one location, to assist surgeons in their explanation to the patient during the consent process

For each specific surgical procedure the text provides:

- Description and some background of the surgical procedure
- Anatomical points and possible variations
- Estimated Frequencies
- Perspective
- Major Complications

From this, a better understanding of the risks, complications and consequences associated with surgical procedures can hopefully be gained by the clinician for explanation of relevant and appropriate aspects to the patient.

The _Estimated frequency lists are not mean't to be totally comprehensive_ or to contain all of the information that needs to be explained in obtaining informed consent from the patient for a surgical procedure. Indeed, _most of the information is for the surgeon_ or reader only, _not designed for the patient_, however, parts should be selected by the surgeon at their discretion for appropriate explanation to the individual patient in the consent process.

Many patients would not understand or would be confused by the number of potential complications that may be associated with a specific surgical procedure, so ***some degree of selective discussion of the risks, complications and consequences would be necessary and advisable,*** as would usually occur in clinical practice. This judgement should necessarily be left to the surgeon, surgeon-in-training or other practitioner.

Preface

Over the last decade or so we have witnessed a rapid change in the consumer demand for information by patients preparing for a surgical procedure. This is fuelled by multiple factors including the 'internet revolution', altered public consumer attitudes, professional patient advocacy, freedom of information laws, insurance issues, risk management, and medicolegal claims made through the legal system throughout the western world, so that the need has arisen for a higher, fairer and clearer standard of *'informed consent'*.

One of the my main difficulties encountered as a young intern, and later as a surgical resident, registrar and consultant surgeon, was obtaining information for use for the pre-operative consenting of patients, and for managing patients on the ward after surgical operations. I watched others struggle with the same problem too. The literature contained many useful facts and clinical studies, but it was unwieldy and very time-consuming to access, and the information that was obtained seemed specific to well-defined studies of highly specific groups of patients. These patient studies, while useful, often did not address my particular patient under treatment in the clinic, operating theatre or ward. Often the studies came from centres with vast experience of a particular condition treated with one type of surgical procedure, constituting a series or trial.

What I wanted to know was:

- The **main complications** associated with a surgical procedure;
- **Information that could be provided** during the consent process, and
- How to **reduce the relative risks** of a complication, where possible

This information was difficult to find in one place!

As a young surgeon, on a very long flight from Adelaide to London, with much time to think and fuelled by some very pleasant champagne, I started making some notes about how I might tackle this problem. My first draft was idle scribble, as I listed the ways surgical complications could be classified. After finding over 10 different classification systems for listing complications, the task became much larger and more complex. I then realized why someone had not taken on this job before!

After a brief in-flight sleep and another glass, the task became far less daunting and suddenly much clearer – the champagne was very good, and there was little else to do in any case!

It was then that I decided to speak with as many of my respected colleagues as I could from around the globe, to get their opinions and advice. The perspectives that emerged were remarkable, as many of them had faced the same dilemmas in their own practices and hospitals, also without a satisfactory solution.

What developed was a composite documentation of information (i) from the published literature and (ii) from the opinions of many experienced surgical practitioners in the field – to provide a text to supply information on **Complications, Risks and Consequences of Surgery** for surgical and other clinical practitioners to use at the bedside and in the clinic.

This work represents the culmination of more than 10 years work with the support and help of colleagues from around the world, for the benefit of their students, junior surgical colleagues, peers, and patients. To them, I owe much gratitude for their cooperation, advice, intellect, experience, wise counsel, friendship and help, for their time, and for their continued encouragement in this rather long-term and complex project. I have already used the text material myself with good effect and it has helped me enormously in my surgical practice.

The text aims to provide health professionals with useful information, which can be selectively used to better inform patients of the potential surgical complications, risks and consequences. I sincerely hope it fulfils this role.

Adelaide, SA, Australia   Brendon J. Coventry, BMBS, PhD,
                                                              FRACS, FACS, FRSM

Acknowledgments

I wish to thank:

The many learned friends and experienced colleagues who have contributed in innumerable ways along the way in the writing of this text.

Professor Sir Peter Morris, formerly Professor of Surgery at Oxford University, and also Past-President of the College of Surgeons of England, for allowing me to base my initial work at the Nuffield Department of Surgery (NDS) and John Radcliffe Hospital in the University of Oxford, for the UK sector of the studies. He and his colleagues have provided encouragement and valuable discussion time over the course of the project.

The (late) Professor John Farndon, Professor of Surgery at the University of Bristol, Bristol Royal Infirmary, UK; and Professor Robert Mansel, Professor of Surgery at the University of Wales, Cardiff, UK for discussions and valued advice.

Professor Charles Balch, then Professor of Surgery at the Johns Hopkins University, Baltimore, Maryland, USA, and Professor Clifford Ko, from UCLA and American College of Surgeons NSQIP Program, USA, for helpful discussions.

Professor Armando Guiliano, formerly of the John Wayne Cancer Institute, Santa Monica, California, USA for his contributions and valuable discussions.

Professor Jonathan Meakins, then Professor of Surgery at McGill University, Quebec, Canada, who provided helpful discussions and encouragement, during our respective sabbatical periods, which coincided in Oxford; and later as Professor of Surgery at Oxford University.

Over the last decade, numerous clinicians have discussed and generously contributed their experience to the validation of the range and relative frequency of complications associated with the wide spectrum of surgical procedures. These clinicians include:

Los Angeles, USA: Professor Carmack Holmes, Cardiothoracic Surgeon, Los Angeles (UCLA); Professor Donald Morton, Melanoma Surgeon, Los Angeles; Dr R Essner, Melanoma Surgeon, Los Angeles.

New York, USA: Professor Murray Brennan; Dr David Jacques; Prof L Blumgart; Dr Dan Coit; Dr Mary Sue Brady (Surgeons, Department of Surgery, Memorial Sloan-Kettering Cancer Centre, New York);

Oxford, UK: Dr Linda Hands, Vascular Surgeon; Dr Jack Collin, Vascular Surgeon; Professor Peter Friend, Transplant and Vascular Surgeon; Dr Nick Maynard, Upper Gastrointestinal Surgeon; Dr Mike Greenall, Breast Surgeon; Dr Jane Clark, Breast Surgeon; Professor Derek Gray, Vascular/Pancreatic Surgeon; Dr Julian Britton, Hepato-Biliary Surgeon; Dr Greg Sadler, Endocrine Surgeon; Dr Christopher Cunningham, Colorectal Surgeon; Professor Neil Mortensen, Colorectal Surgeon; Dr Bruce George, Colorectal Surgeon; Dr Chris Glynn, Anaesthetist (National Health Service (NHS), Oxford, UK).

Bristol, UK: Professor Derek Alderson.

Adelaide, Australia: Professor Guy Ludbrook, Anesthetist; Dr Elizabeth Tam, Anesthetist.

A number of senior medical students at the University of Adelaide, including Hwee Sim Tan, Adelaine S Lam, Ramon Pathi, Mohd Azizan Ghzali, William Cheng, Sue Min Ooi, Teena Silakong, and Balaji Rajacopalin, who assisted during their student projects in the preliminary feasibility studies and research, and their participation is much appreciated. Thanks also to numerous sixth year students, residents and surgeons at Hospitals in Adelaide who participated in questionnaires and surveys.

The support of the University of Adelaide, especially the Department of Surgery, and Royal Adelaide Hospital has been invaluable in allowing the sabbatical time to engineer the collaborations necessary for this project to progress. I thank Professors Glyn Jamieson and Guy Maddern for their support in this regard.

I especially thank the Royal Australasian College of Surgeons for part-support through the Marjorie Hooper Fellowship.

I thank my clinical colleagues on the Breast, Endocrine and Surgical Oncology Unit at the Royal Adelaide Hospital, especially Grantley Gill, James Kollias and Melissa Bochner, for caring for my patients and assuming greater clinical load when I have been away.

Professor Bill Runciman, Australian Patient Safety Foundation, for all of his advice and support; Professors Cliff Hughes and Bruce Barraclough, from the Royal Australasian College of Surgeons, the Clinical Excellence Commission, New South Wales, and the Australian Commission (Council) on Safety and Quality in Healthcare.

Thanks too to Kai Holt, Anne-Marie Bennett and Carrie Cooper who assisted and helped to organise my work. I also acknowledge my collaborator Martin Ashdown for being so patient during distractions from our scientific research work. Also to Graeme Cogdell, Imagart Design Ltd, Adelaide, for his expertise and helpful discussions.

I particularly thank Melissa Morton and her global team at Springer-Verlag for their work in preparing the manuscript for publication.

Importantly, I truly appreciate and thank my wife Christine, my four children and our parents/ wider family for their support in every way towards seeing this project through to its completion, and in believing so much in me, and in my work.

Adelaide, SA, Australia   Brendon J. Coventry, BMBS, PhD,
                                                                              FRACS, FACS, FRSM

Contents

Contributors

Brendon J. Coventry, BMBS, PhD, FRACS, FACS, FRSM Discipline of Surgery, Royal Adelaide Hospital, University of Adelaide, Adelaide, SA, Australia

Clifford Y. Ko, MD, MS, MSHS Division of Research and Optimal Patient Care, American College of Surgeons, Chicago, IL, USA

Villis Marshall, MD, FRACS Department of Surgery, The University of Adelaide, Royal Adelaide Hospital, Adelaide, Australia

David Wattchow, BM, BS, PhD, FRACS Department of Surgery, Flinders Medical Centre, Bedford Park, Australia

Bruce Waxman, BMedSc, MBBS, FRACS, FRCS(Eng), FACS Academic Surgical Unit, Monash University, Monash Health and Southern Clinical School, Dandenong, VIC, Australia

Chapter 1
Introduction

Brendon J. Coventry

This volume deals with complications, risks, and consequences related to a range of procedures under the broad headings of colorectal surgery, anal surgery, perineal surgery, and penile and scrotal surgery.

Important Note

It should be emphasized that the risks and frequencies that are given here *represent derived figures*. These *figures are best estimates of relative frequencies across most institutions*, not merely the highest-performing ones, and as such are often representative of a number of studies, which include different patients with differing comorbidities and different surgeons. In addition, the risks of complications in lower- or higher-risk patients may lie outside these estimated ranges, and individual clinical judgment is required as to the expected risks communicated to the patient and staff or for other purposes. The range of risks is also derived from experience and the literature; while risks outside this range may exist, certain risks may be reduced or absent due to variations of procedures or surgical approaches. It is recognized that different patients, practitioners, institutions, regions, and countries may vary in their requirements and recommendations.

Individual clinical judgment should always be exercised, of course, when applying the general information contained in these documents to individual patients in a clinical setting.

The authors would like to thank Professor Neil Mortensen, Oxford, United Kingdom, who as an experienced clinician discussed the chapters and acted as an advisor.

B.J. Coventry, BMBS, PhD, FRACS, FACS, FRSM
Discipline of Surgery, Royal Adelaide Hospital, University of Adelaide,
L5 Eleanor Harrald Building, North Terrace, 5000 Adelaide, SA, Australia
e-mail: brendon.coventry@adelaide.edu.au

B.J. Coventry (ed.), *Lower Abdominal and Perineal Surgery*,
Surgery: Complications, Risks and Consequences,
DOI 10.1007/978-1-4471-5469-3_1, © Springer-Verlag London 2014

Chapter 2
Colorectal Surgery

Bruce Waxman, Brendon J. Coventry, David Wattchow, and Clifford Ko

General Perspective and Overview

The relative risks and complications increase proportionately according to the site of resection and anastomosis within the colon/rectum from cecum to the anus. This is principally related to the surgical accessibility, ability to reduce tension, blood supply, risk of tissue injury, hematoma formation, and technical ease of achieving anastomosis. Photographs that illustrate various aspects of colorectal surgery are shown in Figs. 2.1 and 2.2.

The main serious complication is **anastomotic leakage,** which can be minimized by the adequate colonic mobilization, reduction of tension, and ensuring satisfactory blood supply to the bowel. Avoidance of twisting or obstruction of bowel, either at the anastomosis or ileostomy, is imperative. The anastomosis can be tested in a variety of ways, including with air or povidone-iodine, so a small leak can be detected intraoperatively and sutured. Infection is the main sequel of anastomotic leakage or hematoma formation and may lead to **abscess formation, peritonitis,**

B. Waxman, BMedSc, MBBS, FRACS, FRCS(Eng), FACS (✉)
Academic Surgical Unit, Monash University, Monash Health
and Southern Clinical School, Dandenong, VIC, Australia
e-mail: bruce.waxman@southernhealth.org.au

B.J. Coventry, BMBS, PhD, FRACS, FACS, FRSM
Discipline of Surgery, Royal Adelaide Hospital, University of Adelaide,
L5 Eleanor Harrald Building, North Terrace, 5000 Adelaide, SA, Australia

D. Wattchow, BM, BS, PhD, FRACS
Department of Surgery, Flinders Medical Centre, Bedford Park, SA, Australia

C. Ko, MD, MS, MSHS
Division of Research and Optimal Patient Care, American College of Surgeons,
Chicago, IL, USA

Department of Colorectal Surgery, University of California,
Los Angeles, USA

B.J. Coventry (ed.), *Lower Abdominal and Perineal Surgery*,
Surgery: Complications, Risks and Consequences,
DOI 10.1007/978-1-4471-5469-3_2, © Springer-Verlag London 2014

Fig. 2.1 Infected wound
post-colonic resection

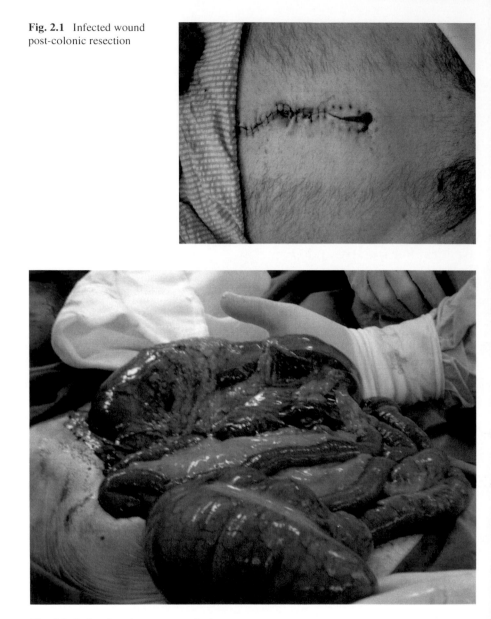

Fig. 2.2 Ischemic colon post-op volvulus

and **systemic sepsis**. **Multi-system failure** and **death** remain serious potential complications of colonic surgery and systemic infection.

   Loop ileostomies are infrequently used for anastomoses proximal to the sigmoid colon, but are often used for low rectal anastomoses to reduce anastomotic pressure during healing. Reversal of the loop ileostomy can be performed 3–6 months later in many cases. Stomas are associated with separate complications also. Increasingly, **colonic pouches** are used for very low anastomoses to recreate the rectum and provide a longer-term reservoir function. Despite all these maneuvers, low rectal anastomoses still have a higher overall leak rate and mortality than standard colonic anastomoses.

The risk of **bowel, bladder**, and **sexual dysfunction** increases with proximity of colorectal resection to the pelvis and is almost exclusively associated with lower rectal surgery. Technical refinements, like meso-rectal dissection with preservation of the hypogastric nerves, depending on tumor involvement, can reduce disability significantly. The introduction of robotic-assisted laparoscopic surgery, with better visualization and improved tissue dissection, may further reduce the incidence of nerve injury but with a considerable increase in economic cost. Rectal, bladder, and sexual sensation may be altered, and rectal surgery may be associated with more **frequent bowel actions and reduced control**, all of which may recover partially or completely over the months postoperatively.

Positioning on the operating table has been associated with increased risk of **deep venous thrombosis** and **nerve palsies**, especially in prolonged procedures. With the modified Lloyd-Davies position, especially if placed in the steep Trendelenburg position, **limb ischemia, compartment syndrome**, and **common peroneal nerve palsy** are recognized potential complications, which should be checked for, as the patient's position may change during surgery.

Mortality associated with colorectal procedures ranged from 4.4 % to 6.5 % overall (30-day perioperative mortality); however, in a study of 11,036 patients (1987–1996), this varied from 3.7 % for elective to 11.2 % for emergency procedures. Variation for the type of procedure also occurred from 6.9 % for right hemicolectomy and 8.6 % for left hemicolectomy to 3.8 % for anterior resection.

With these factors and facts in mind, the information given in these chapters must be appropriately and discernibly interpreted and used.

The **use of specialized colorectal surgery units with standardized preoperative assessment, multidisciplinary input, and high-quality postoperative care** is essential to the success of complex colorectal surgery overall and can significantly reduce risk of complications or aid early detection, prompt intervention, and cost. Furthermore, there is evidence that high-volume surgery units have better outcomes than low-volume units particularly for low rectal surgery.

Important Note

It should be emphasized that the risks and frequencies that are given here *represent derived figures*. These *figures are best estimates of relative frequencies across most institutions*, not merely the highest-performing ones, and as such are often representative of a number of studies, which include different patients with differing comorbidities and different surgeons. In addition, the risks of complications in lower- or higher-risk patients may lie outside these estimated ranges, and individual clinical judgment is required as to the expected risks communicated to the patient and staff or for other purposes. The range of risks is also derived from experience and the literature; while risks outside this range may exist, certain risks may be reduced or absent due to variations of procedures or surgical approaches. It is recognized that different patients, practitioners, institutions, regions, and countries may vary in their requirements and recommendations.

Rigid Sigmoidoscopy and/or Rectal Biopsy

Description

This can be performed without anesthesia as an office procedure or under general anesthesia at initiation of a colorectal procedure to define the level of a rectal lesion, during examination of the anorectal region under anesthesia, and at the time of routine surgery for benign anal conditions (e.g., hemorrhoidectomy, fissure-in-ano) to check for any pathology in the lower rectum. The objective is to examine the rectum into the lower sigmoid colon up to 25 cm to define any lesion(s) and perhaps biopsy these. Preferably the patient would have been prepared with an enema to clear the rectum.

The procedure is best performed by an experienced surgeon, with an assistant or a nurse, with a long suction catheter and biopsy forceps available.

Rigid sigmoidoscopy may also be used to decompress a sigmoid volvulus. This may be performed either on the patient's bed or on the operating table, and it is essential that adequate preparation is given in anticipation of large volumes of feculent fluid coming through the sigmoidoscope. The availability of suction and a rectal tube is mandatory.

Anatomical Points

The anorectal anatomy is usually constant but can be altered by abscesses, sepsis, fissure, fistula, rectal tumors, pelvic pathology, and sigmoid colon pathology, including diverticular disease, strictures, volvulus, intussusception, and tumors. The lower rectum is directed backwards, the mid-rectum upwards, and then the upper rectum forwards.

Perspective

See Table 2.1. Rectal perforation is the most serious complication. This may be either extraperitoneal or intraperitoneal and should be recognized by the operator as a tear associated with bleeding. This most commonly occurs when an inexperienced operator is performing the procedure, when undue force is used, or when the rectum or sigmoid is fixed by either a tumor or an inflammatory process. Extraperitoneal perforation may not require any surgery, whereas intraperitoneal perforation is more serious and may require colonic defunctioning for diversion of the fecal stream. The risk of perforation from colonoscopy is approximately double

Table 2.1 Rigid sigmoidoscopy (and/or rectal biopsy) estimated frequency of complications, risks, and consequences

Complications, risks, and consequences	Estimated frequency
Most significant/serious complications	
Bleeding without biopsy (major)	0.1–1 %
Bleeding with biopsy (major)	5–20 %
Missed pathology[a]	1–5 %
Rare significant/serious problems	
Perforation[a]	0.1–1 %
Infection	0.1–1 %
Less serious complications	
Discomfort	>80 %

[a]Dependent on underlying pathology, anatomy, surgical technique, and preferences

that from sigmoidoscopy. Hemorrhage following biopsy may also occur and is more likely to occur in biopsying normal rectal mucosa than biopsying tumors. Overall, infection is rare, but perineal necrotizing fasciitis or Fournier's gangrene is reported. Discomfort from insufflation of gas or instrument insertion is common, and the patient should be warned of this.

Major Complications

Major complications are very rare. The procedure is usually very straightforward. **Rectal tears** and/or **bowel perforation** may rarely occur, potentially leading to **local sepsis, abscess formation**, and sometimes **systemic sepsis** and very rarely **multi-system organ failure. Bleeding** may be severe especially after biopsy, sometimes associated with anticoagulant therapy or bleeding diatheses. Particular care should be taken in immunosuppressed patients, those with ulcerative colitis and carcinoma, following radiation therapy and rectosigmoid tethering, or where vision is obscured by blood or feces. The need for **general anesthesia** and **further surgery** is possible if a severe injury occurs and requires diversion colostomy/ileostomy and/or repair.

Consent and Risk Reduction

Main Points to Explain

- Discomfort
- Bleeding
- Perforation

Colonoscopy (Including Flexible Sigmoidoscopy or Endoscopy of the Rectum and Left Colon)

Description

This procedure is ideally performed under general anesthesia or IV sedation in the presence of a qualified anesthetist for adequate monitoring. This provides the patient with adequate relaxation, analgesia, and the ability for the assistant to aid the endoscopist in providing pressure or changing the posture of the patient from lateral to lithotomy or even to prone position while maintaining the airway. Occasionally, no anesthesia is required. Preoperative preparation of the bowel is mandatory to provide adequate views and to reduce the chances of complication.

Anatomical Points

The basic anatomy of the anus, rectum, and colon is relatively constant; however, the length and tortuosity of various sections of the colon (notably the sigmoid and transverse colon) may vary considerably. The cecum may also be very mobile. The hepatic and splenic flexures and sigmoid loop may be tethered and make negotiation with the colonoscope difficult.

Perspective

See Table 2.2. Colonoscopy in experienced hands is a relatively safe procedure. However, because perforation is such a significant complication, the informed consent process is vital so that the patient has full understanding of the risks.

The risks of perforation are significantly increased when therapeutic endoscopy is performed using either the "hot biopsy" technique or the snare and diathermy technique. Therapeutic biopsy-related perforations are more likely in the right colon, and perforation associated with diagnostic colonoscopy is more likely in the left colon, particularly in the sigmoid. The overall risk of perforation is about 1:1,000.

Early recognition and aggressive management of perforations following flexible endoscopy is vital to reduce long-term septic complications. Extraperitoneal perforations are usually less serious but may require antibiotics in addition to careful observation, whereas intraperitoneal perforation may require surgical intervention, including laparotomy and colostomy or ileostomy to divert the fecal stream in some cases, with or without resection or oversewing of the perforation site. The risk of perforation from colonoscopy is approximately double that from sigmoidoscopy.

Table 2.2 Colonoscopy estimated frequency of complications, risks, and consequences

Complications, risks, and consequences	Estimated frequency
Most significant/serious complications	
Failure to visualize parts of colon[a,b]	1–5 %
Bleeding/hematoma formation (major)	0.1–1 %
Perforation[a,b]	0.1–1 %
Laparotomy	0.1–1 %
Infection	0.1–1 %
Rare significant/serious problems	
Aspiration pneumonitis[a]	0.1–1 %
Hypoxia[a]	0.1–1 %
Multi-system failure (renal, pulmonary, cardiac failure)[b]	<0.1 %
Less serious complications	
Gas bloating (transient)	50–80 %
Paralytic ileus	5–20 %
Injury to hemorrhoids[a]	1–5 %
From purgative bowel preparation	
From colonoscope	
Glutaraldehyde[a]	
Subcutaneous emphysema/pneumothorax/pneumomediastinum	0.1–1 %
Traumatic anal fissure[a]	0.1–1 %
Pain and discomfort[a]	5–20 %

[a]Risks and complications that should be avoidable with particular safety measures
[b]Dependent on underlying pathology, anatomy, surgical technique, and preferences

Bleeding is rarely severe, but a small amount of bleeding after biopsy is not uncommon.

Major Complications

Colonoscopy is usually a straightforward procedure. Major complications are rare but include full-thickness **perforation of the rectum or colon**, which can require **further surgery** (laparotomy or per-anal procedure). Local **infection, abscess formation, fistula, systemic sepsis, and multi-system organ failure** may follow perforation. Particular care should be taken in immunosuppressed patients, those with ulcerative colitis and carcinoma, following radiation therapy and rectosigmoid tethering, or where vision is obscured by blood or feces. **Hypoxia** from sedation is rare, and brain damage exceedingly rare with the use of oxygen monitors and an anesthetist supervising. **Severe bleeding** is uncommon, but can rarely require **blood transfusion** or further surgery. **Failure to diagnose** is possible, and **inability to complete the full colonoscopy** is not uncommon, related to the anatomy, previous surgery, bowel preparation, and experience of the colonoscopist. A **repeat colonoscopy** or another method may be required. Although rare, **aspiration pneumonitis** can be a serious and lethal complication but is reduced by an adequate fasting period and good airway management.

Consent and Risk Reduction

Main Points to Explain

- Discomfort and gas bloating
- Bleeding
- Problems with sedation
- Failure to visualize parts of the colon
- Perforation
- Infection
- Further surgery: laparotomy

Open Appendectomy

Description

General anesthesia is used. The patient is positioned in the supine position and is best examined when anesthetized to assess whether there is a mass to determine the best site for the incision. Rectal examination under anesthesia may be useful to assess the presence of any pelvic mass particularly in the female.

The objective of the operation is to perform removal of the appendix and also to examine the pelvis for pelvic pathology, particularly in the female, and the terminal ileum for the presence of a Meckel's diverticulum or other pathology causing local peritonitis, particularly if the appendix appears normal. Occasionally, the inflammatory process, phlegmon or abscess, is so extensive that the appendix cannot be removed, and it may be judicious to simply drain the abscess.

Under most circumstances the appendix can be removed using a transverse (Lanz) skin incision and a muscle splitting incision of the internal oblique and transversus muscles. When other pathology is encountered, either Crohn's disease affecting the terminal ileum and cecum, diverticular disease affecting the sigmoid colon or cecum, or an abscess involving the right fallopian tube, ovary, and uterus, the incision may be extended or an alternative midline incision performed.

The surgical approach in open appendectomy is a paradox in that it disobeys the primary principle of abdominal surgery that being adequate access and exposure. A small incision is often made to obtain a good cosmetic result, making access more difficult. Surgeons should never hesitate to increase the length of the skin incision and divide the abdominal muscles to provide better access to the peritoneal cavity.

Under these circumstances, the cecum should be mobilized by dividing the congenital adhesions to bring the cecum well into the wound to show the display and full length of the appendix, particularly its junction with the cecum.

Anatomical Points

The appendix origin lies at the confluence of the taenia coli; however, its tip can vary enormously in position, lying retrocecally (~75 % cases), pelvic (20 %), or retro-ileal/pre-ileal (5 %). The length of the appendix varies also and can reach the upper ascending colon posteriorly. The appendix and cecum may enter a large inguinal hernia sac. An inflamed appendix, if retrocecal or pelvic in location, may irritate the ureter. Hematuria or dysuria may occur. Irritation of the bladder or colon can cause urinary urgency and/or diarrhea. Irritation of the psoas muscle by an inflamed retrocecal appendix or abscess may cause hip discomfort on movement. Maldescent of the appendix is rare, due to malrotation of the cecum, which remains high in the hepatic region. Agenesis, duplication, and situs inversus (L-side appendix) are exceedingly rare but can occur.

Perspective

See Table 2.3. Infective complications are the most common following appendectomy, wound infection being the most significant. This may be minimized by adequate exposure, preoperative prophylactic antibiotics, and copious lavage of the abdominal cavity and the wound with large volumes of warm saline.

In grossly contaminated (dirty) wounds, drainage of the pelvis and wound, delayed primary skin closure, or the use of gauze pledgets impregnated with antiseptic may be used in an effort to reduce risk of infection. The other option is to leave the skin wound open and use vacuum-assisted dressings.

Abscess formation can occur in the pelvis, right paracolic gutter, between loops of small bowel, or occasionally subphrenic space, but are uncommon. Damage to anatomical structures in the region may occur, particularly the ilioinguinal or iliohypogastric nerves as they traverse close to the incision or the inferior epigastric vessels. Right inguinal hernia and right femoral hernia are more common after appendectomy.

Different techniques of dealing with the appendix stump can avoid complications associated with the stump including intraperitoneal abscess, "recurrent" appendicitis, and fecal fistula from breakdown of the wound closure of the cecum. Moreover, long-term complications of small bowel obstructions with adhesions either to the appendix base or to the aperture of the appendix mesentery can occur. Inversion of the stump has been associated with increased risk of small bowel obstruction. Firm suture transfixion/ligation of the appendix base against the cecum

Table 2.3 Open appendectomy estimated frequency of complications, risks, and consequences

Complications, risks, and consequences	Estimated frequency
Most significant/serious complications	
Infection[a]	5–20 %
Subcutaneous	5–20 %
Intraabdominal/pelvic (peritonitis, abscess)	0.1–1 %
Systemic sepsis	0.1–1 %
Hepatic portal sepsis (rare)	<0.1 %
Bleeding/hematoma formation[a]	
Wound	1–5 %
Intraabdominal	0.1–1 %
Extension of wound for access/safety (for improving exposure)[a]	1–5 %
Midline laparotomy (possibility if other pathology found)[a]	0.1–1 %
Rare significant/serious problems	
Multi-system failure (renal, pulmonary, cardiac failure)	0.1–1 %
Small bowel obstruction (early or late)[a]	0.1–1 %
[Anastomotic stenosis/adhesion formation]	
Deep venous thrombosis	0.1–1 %
Inguinal hernia (right side)	0.1–1 %
Fecal fistula[a]	<0.1 %
Ureteric injury (v. rare)[a]	<0.1 %
Vascular injury (v. rare)[a]	<0.1 %
Less serious complications	
Paralytic ileus	50–80 %
Nerve paresthesia	0.1– %1
Iliohypogastric/ilioinguinal nerve	
Seroma formation	0.1–1 %
Incisional hernia (delayed heavy lifting/straining for 8 weeks)	0.1–1 %
Pain/tenderness [wound pain]	
Acute (<4 weeks)	>80 %
Chronic (>12 weeks)	1–5 %
Nasogastric tube[a]	1–5 %
Wound scarring (poor cosmesis/wound deformity)[a]	1–5 %
Wound drain tube(s)[a]	1–5 %

[a]Dependent on underlying pathology, anatomy, surgical technique, and preferences

usually avoids appendix stump complications. Complete appendectomy with transection of the appendix flush with the cecum and closure in two layers with a monofilament absorbable suture will eliminate an appendix stump.

Major Complications

Serious complications are **abscess formation, fistula or sinus formation**, and **systemic sepsis**, which may rarely lead to **multi-system organ failure** and even mortality. Early surgery and preoperative antibiotics have reduced these complications significantly. Preexisting comorbidities including age, established generalized peritonitis, and immunosuppression can increase risk of infection greatly. **Wound infection** may be reduced by delaying skin closure for several days. Further surgery may be warranted. **Severe bleeding** is rare, and transfusion uncommon. Concealed postoperative bleeding is rare. Persistent **wound sinuses** or a **fecal fistula** requires prolonged hospitalization and dressings but most close within 2 months. **Prolonged ileus** and later (even decades later) **small bowel obstruction** can occur, but are surprisingly uncommon even with extensive adhesions. The possibility of a **laparotomy** and even a **colostomy** should be mentioned, should other pathology be found, although uncommon. **Nerve injury**, either at surgery or later scar adhesions, can cause severe discomfort and rarely chronic pain problems. **Incisional hernia formation** is more common after wound infection and/or dehiscence. **Ureteric injury** or **iliac arterial injury** is exceedingly rare, although reported, but can be catastrophic.

Consent and Risk Reduction

Main Points to Explain

- GA risk
- Wound infection
- Abscess formation
- Bleeding
- Further surgery: laparotomy

Laparoscopic Appendectomy

Description

General anesthetic is used. The patient is positioned in the supine position and is best examined when anesthetized to assess whether there is a mass to determine the best site for the incision. Rectal examination under anesthesia may be useful to assess the presence of any pelvic mass. Some surgeons prefer the modified Lloyd-Davies position.

The objective of the operation is to perform removal of the appendix, using the principles of minimal invasive surgery, and should include laparoscopic examination of the peritoneal cavity to examine the pelvis for pelvic pathology, particularly in the female, and the terminal ileum for the presence of a Meckel's diverticulum or other pathology causing local peritonitis, particularly if the appendix appears normal. Occasionally, the inflammatory process, phlegmon or abscess, is so extensive that the appendix cannot be removed and it may be judicious to simply drain the abscess.

When other pathology is encountered, either Crohn's disease affecting the terminal ileum and cecum, diverticular disease affecting the sigmoid colon or cecum, or an abscess involving the right fallopian tube, ovary, and uterus, an alternative approach and open surgery may be preferred.

Surgeons should never hesitate to convert to an open incision if the safety of the operation is jeopardized through increased risk of injury, progress is poor, or vision is inadequate.

Anatomical Points

The appendix origin lies at the confluence of the taenia coli; however, its tip can vary enormously in position, lying retrocecally (~75 % cases), pelvic (20 %), or retro-ileal/pre-ileal (5 %). The length of the appendix varies also and can reach the upper ascending colon posteriorly. The appendix and cecum may enter a large inguinal hernia sac. An inflamed appendix, if retrocecal or pelvic in location, may irritate the ureter. Hematuria or dysuria may occur. Irritation of the bladder or colon can cause urinary urgency and/or diarrhea. Irritation of the psoas muscle by an inflamed retrocecal appendix or abscess may cause hip discomfort on movement. Maldescent of the appendix is rare, due to malrotation of the cecum, which remains high in the hepatic region. Agenesis, duplication, and situs inversus (L side appendix) are exceedingly rare but can occur.

Perspective

See Table 2.4. Infective complications are the most common following appendectomy, wound infection being the most frequent. Use of a bag to collect and contain the appendix for removal may reduce risk of infection. Adequate exposure, good port placement, preoperative prophylactic antibiotics, and copious lavage of the abdominal cavity and the wounds with large volumes of warm saline may also assist. In grossly contaminated (dirty) wounds, drainage of the pelvis and wound, delayed primary skin closure, or the use of gauze pledgets impregnated with antiseptic may be used in an effort to reduce risk of infection. Abscess formation can occur in the pelvis, right paracolic gutter, between loops of small bowel, or occasionally subphrenic space, but are uncommon. Gas embolism is associated with Veress needle insertion, which can be virtually eliminated by open cutdown methods. Similarly, injury to the bladder, bowel, or vessels during port insertion can usually be avoided by open cutdown insertion methods. Emptying the bladder is mandatory before port placement. Pneumothorax is a rare, idiosyncratic complication, probably from diaphragmatic leakage of gas.

Table 2.4 Laparoscopic appendectomy estimated frequency of complications, risks, and consequences

Complications, risks, and consequences	Estimated frequency
Most significant/serious complications	
Infection[a]	5–20 %
Subcutaneous	5–20 %
Intraabdominal/pelvic (peritonitis, abscess)	0.1–1 %
Systemic sepsis	0.1–1 %
Hepatic portal sepsis (rare)	<0.1 %
Port site	0.1–1 %
Bleeding/hematoma formation[a]	
Wound	1–5 %
Intraabdominal	0.1–1 %
Conversion to open operation	1–5 %
Midline laparotomy (possibility if other pathology found)[a]	0.1–1 %
Rare significant/serious problems	
Injury to the bowel or blood vessels (trocar or diathermy)	0.1–1 %
Duodenal/gastric/small bowel/colonic	
Gas embolus	0.1–1 %
Multi-system failure (renal, pulmonary, cardiac failure)	0.1–1 %
Small bowel obstruction (early or late)[a]	0.1–1 %
[Anastomotic stenosis/adhesion formation]	
Deep venous thrombosis	0.1–1 %
Inguinal hernia (right side)	0.1–1 %
Extension of wound for access/safety (for improving exposure)[a]	1–5 %
Fecal fistula[a]	
Ureteric injury[a]	<0.1 %
Vascular injury[a]	<0.1 %
Less serious complications	
Paralytic ileus	50–80 %
Nerve paresthesia	0.1–1 %
Iliohypogastric/ilioinguinal nerve	
Seroma formation	0.1–1 %
Pain/tenderness [wound pain]	
Acute (<4 weeks)	>80 %
Chronic (>12 weeks)	1–5 %
Port site hernia formation	0.1–1 %
Wound scarring (poor cosmesis/wound deformity)[a]	1–5 %
Nasogastric tube[a]	1–5 %
Wound drain tube(s)[a]	1–5 %

[a]Dependent on underlying pathology, anatomy, surgical technique, and preferences

Major Complications

Abscess formation, fistula or sinus formation, and **systemic sepsis** are serious complications that may rarely lead to **multi-system organ failure** and even mortality. Early surgery and preoperative antibiotics have reduced these complications significantly. Preexisting comorbidities including age, established generalized peritonitis, and immunosuppression can increase risk of infection greatly. **Wound infection** may be reduced by delaying skin closure for several days. Further surgery may be warranted. **Severe bleeding** is rare, and transfusion uncommon. Concealed postoperative bleeding is rare. Persistent **wound sinuses** or a **fecal fistula** requires prolonged hospitalization and dressings but most close within 2 months. **Prolonged ileus** and later (even decades later) **small bowel obstruction** can occur, but are surprisingly uncommon even with extensive adhesions. The possibility of a **laparotomy**, and even a **colostomy** should be mentioned, if other pathology is found, although uncommon. **Nerve injury**, either at surgery or later scar adhesions, can cause severe discomfort and rarely chronic pain problems. **Gas embolism** is a very rare but catastrophic complication. **Incisional hernia formation** is more common after wound infection and/or dehiscence. **Ureteric injury** or **iliac arterial injury** is exceedingly rare but can be catastrophic.

Consent and Risk Reduction

Main Points to Explain

- GA risk
- Wound infection
- Abscess formation
- Bleeding
- Risks of laparoscopy
- Conversion to open surgery
- Further surgery

Colostomy and Mucous Fistula (Including Laparotomy)

Description

General anesthetic is used. The patient is often best positioned in the modified Lloyd-Davies position with a urinary catheter in the bladder. This provides access to the anus and rectum, should this be required, and also provides access for the scrubbed nurse during the operation or the surgeon to gain easier access to the left upper quadrant particularly to perform mobilization of the splenic flexure. Preoperative sitting, ideally by a stomal therapy nurse, is highly recommended.

Colostomy and mucous fistula is most often performed with colonic resection, where conditions mitigate against performing a primary anastomosis or where subtotal colectomy with ileorectal anastomosis is contraindicated. To make the later second stage of the procedure, viz., colo-colonic anastomosis, more straightforward, it is best that the proximal colon and distal colon are brought out through the same aperture. Ideally, the site of the stoma is planned before the operation commences. In an emergency setting, this is not possible, and the aperture of the stoma is best placed in a horizontal plane, along a line from the umbilicus to the anterior superior iliac spine, approximately 3–4 cm lateral to the umbilicus usually on the left side. The stoma should ideally go through the rectus muscle. It is important to align the fascia/muscle/skin openings so as not to "scissor" the opening which can cause outlet obstruction. Designing the correct sized opening for the bowel caliber is vital to avoid narrowing due to a too small opening or prolapse/hernia due to a too large opening. The pathology, degree of bowel edema, and anatomical location (e.g., colon vs. ileum) can influence this at the time of surgery.

The abdomen is closed and the stomata are fashioned together at the skin surface using absorbable suture material.

Anatomical Points

The colon length and mobility may vary considerably. This may be partially determined by the peritoneal attachments and adhesions from previous surgery or inflammation. The mesenteric length may also vary, often shortened by disease processes, such as diverticular disease. Intraperitoneal, extraperitoneal, and body wall fat may also limit the ability to raise bowel to the skin easily. Thick abdominal muscle may tend to constrict the stoma.

Perspective

See Table 2.5. Relief of obstruction and control of infection usually make major complications infrequent, and complications are often minor in nature. Without surgery, consequences are usually dire. Ischemia of the colostomy in the immediate postoperative period is the most serious complication and can be best avoided by making the aperture of adequate size and ensuring arterial blood supply to the proximal cut end of the colon. Because the colostomy is fashioned after abdominal closure, it is vital to ensure adequate length of colon can be brought out through the aperture to create the colostomy. This may require mobilization of the splenic flexure, which would be a mandatory procedure for any resection of the left colon. Retraction of the stoma due to distension is another potential complication due to traction and may also cause ischemia. Fecal leakage is usually avoidable but can occur, leading to infection and abscess formation. Separation of the mucosa and skin may occur particularly in patients with medical comorbidities and malnutrition and when taking medication that may reduce wound healing. The involvement of the stomal therapist in the preoperative and postoperative phases is essential.

Table 2.5 Colostomy and mucous fistula estimated frequency of complications, risks, and consequences

Complications, risks, and consequences	Estimated frequency
Most significant/serious complications	
Infection[a] overall	5–20 %
Subcutaneous	5–20 %
Intraabdominal/pelvic (peritonitis, abscess)	0.1–1 %
Systemic sepsis	0.1–1 %
Hepatic portal sepsis (rare)	<0.1 %
Bleeding/hematoma formation[a]	
Wound	1–5 %
Intraabdominal	0.1–1 %
Retraction of stoma	1–5 %
Parastomal hernia formation	1–5 %
Rare significant/serious problems	
Stomal prolapse	0.1–1 %
Small bowel obstruction (early or late)[a]	0.1–1 %
[Anastomotic stenosis/adhesion formation]	
Misorientation[a]	0.1–1 %
Entero-cutaneous fistula	0.1–1 %
Fecal fistula[a]	0.1–1 %
Ischemic necrosis	0.1–1 %
Wound dehiscence	0.1–1 %
Deep venous thrombosis	0.1–1 %
Ureteric injury (v. rare)[a]	<0.1 %
Vascular injury (v. rare)[a]	<0.1 %
Multi-system failure (renal, pulmonary, cardiac failure)	0.1–1 %
Death[a]	0.1–1 %
Less serious complications	
Paralytic ileus	50–80 %
Seroma formation	0.1–1 %
Stomal ulceration	0.1–1 %
Stomal leakage (poor sealing of bag)	1–5 %
Malpositioning of colostomy	0.1–1 %
Incisional hernia (delayed heavy lifting/straining for 8 weeks)	0.1–1 %
Cutaneous infective sinus (abscess associated)	0.1–1 %
Wound scarring (poor cosmesis/wound deformity)[a]	50–80 %
Pain/tenderness [wound pain]	
Acute (<4 weeks)	>80 %
Chronic (>12 weeks)	1–5 %
Nasogastric tube[a]	1–5 %
Wound drain tube(s)[a]	1–5 %

[a]Dependent on underlying pathology, anatomy, surgical technique, preferences, and experience

Longer-term complications include leakage from stoma from poor appliance fit. Reversal of the double-barreled colostomy is usually desired; however, some circumstances may make this unwise, for example, in elderly and patients with significant comorbidities who are at high risk.

Major Complications

Stomal and colonic ischemia are serious complications of both stomal constriction and tension on the bowel, potentially associated with any devascularization during dissection. These are usually avoidable, or reducible, risks. **Bowel necrosis** and **fecal leakage** are potential consequences, leading to **wound infection** and **peritonitis**, often with **abscess formation** and possibly **fistula formation**. Systemic **sepsis** and consequent **multi-system organ failure** may supervene, both associated with significant morbidity and **mortality**. **Early reoperation for stomal revision** may avoid this. **Ureteric injury** and **vascular injury** are rare, unless a colonic mass is attached to the retroperitoneum and ureter. **Further surgery** at the time and after may then be required. Infection is associated with a greater risk of later **stomal and wound hernia formation**. Local complications such as **fistula formation, cellulitis**, and **external leakage** can be major for the patient and staff.

Consent and Risk Reduction

Main Points to Explain

- GA risk
- Wound infection
- Abscess formation
- Bleeding
- Stoma problems
- Risks of reversal
- Possible injury to blood vessels, bowel, and ureter
- Further surgery

Loop Colostomy

Description

General anesthetic is usually used; however, local or spinal anesthesia may be used for elderly and infirmed patients. The patient is positioned either in supine or in the Lloyd-Davies position (as described above) with a urinary catheter in the bladder. Preoperative sitting, ideally by a stomal therapy nurse, is highly recommended. In an emergency setting, siting the stoma may not be possible, and the aperture of the stoma is best placed in a horizontal plane, in either the right upper quadrant for a transverse colon loop or left lower quadrant for a sigmoid loop. The stoma should ideally go through the rectus muscle.

The objective of this operation is to perform a defunctioning stoma. There is considerable debate as to whether a loop colostomy or a loop ileostomy is a better method of defunctioning, whatever the indication. Many colorectal surgeons prefer loop ileostomy because it preserves the colon and its blood supply, not compromising any future surgery on the colon.

The dilemma is that whereas a loop colostomy is associated with significant complications particularly of prolapse and parastomal hernia, it is associated with fewer complications with the closure. Whereas loop ileostomy has fewer complications of prolapse and parastomal hernia, and often defunctions more efficiently than loop colostomy, there are more significant complications associated with the closure of the loop ileostomy. If a loop colostomy is chosen, obtaining an adequate length of viable colon is mandatory for the success of the stoma. A rod is used to support the loop colostomy in the immediate postoperative period to avoid stomal retraction. Different devices can be used for the rod. A flexible plastic catheter (e.g., FG8 infant feeding tube) is quite useful. The full-length tube can be used to pull the colon out through the aperture and then cut to size, and each end is sutured to the skin with nonabsorbable sutures and removed at ~10 days. It is important to align the fascia/muscle/skin openings so as not to "scissor" the opening which can cause outlet obstruction. Designing the correct sized opening for the bowel caliber is vital to avoid narrowing due to a too small opening or prolapse/hernia due to a too large opening. The pathology, degree of bowel edema, and anatomical location (e.g., transverse vs. sigmoid colon) can influence this at the time of surgery.

Anatomical Points

The transverse colon is often selected in the right upper abdomen, although any mobile section of colon can be used (e.g., sigmoid). The position of the transverse colon may vary considerably, and a plain abdominal x-ray or CT scan may assist in preoperative localization. The stomal site should not be too close to the costal margin or umbilicus to permit better adherence of the stoma bag and reduce leakage. The omentum or small bowel may obscure the colon, and a very redundant (sigmoid) colon or cecum can be confusing, especially if dilated. Adhesions from past surgery can tether the colon and reduce mobility.

Perspective

See Table 2.6. Loop colostomy is usually a straightforward procedure, associated with mainly minor complications, and can effectively defunction the colon and usefully relieve a colonic obstruction. On occasions, the stoma may "valve" and not work well. Ischemia of the stoma in the initial postoperative period is the most significant problem and is avoided by using the principle outlined above. Long-term problems with prolapse and peristomal hernia formation are almost universal with loop colostomy. If a colostomy is chosen as a permanent form of defunctioning,

Table 2.6 Loop colostomy estimated frequency of complications, risks, and consequences

Complications, risks, and consequences	Estimated frequency
Most significant/serious complications	
Infection[a] overall	5–20 %
Subcutaneous	5–20 %
Intraabdominal/pelvic (peritonitis, abscess)	0.1–1 %
Systemic sepsis	0.1–1 %
Hepatic portal sepsis (rare)	<0.1 %
Bleeding/hematoma formation[a]	
Wound	1–5 %
Intraabdominal	0.1–1 %
Retraction of stoma	5–20 %
Rare significant/serious problems	
Stomal prolapse	0.1–1 %
Parastomal hernia formation	0.1–1 %
Small bowel obstruction (early or late)[a]	0.1–1 %
[Anastomotic stenosis/adhesion formation]	
Misorientation[a]	0.1–1 %
Entero-cutaneous fistula	0.1–1 %
Fecal fistula[a]	0.1–1 %
Deep venous thrombosis	0.1–1 %
Ischemic bowel necrosis	<0.1 %
Wound dehiscence	<0.1 %
Multi-system failure (renal, pulmonary, cardiac failure)[a]	0.1–1 %
Death[a]	0.1–1 %
Less serious complications	
Paralytic ileus	1–5 %
Seroma formation	0.1–1 %
Malpositioning of colostomy	0.1–1 %
Stomal leakage (poor sealing of bag)	1–5 %
Stomal ulceration	0.1–1 %
Cutaneous infective sinus (abscess associated)	0.1–1 %
Pain/tenderness [wound pain]	
Acute (<4 weeks)	>80 %
Chronic (>12 weeks)	1–5 %
Incisional hernia (delayed heavy lifting/straining for 8 weeks)	0.1–1 %
Wound scarring (poor cosmesis/wound deformity)[a]	50–80 %
Nasogastric tube[a]	1–5 %
Wound drain tube(s)[a]	1–5 %

[a]Dependent on underlying pathology, anatomy, surgical technique, and preferences

then an end colostomy of the proximal colon and staple closure of the distal colon is probably preferable. If, however, a loop colostomy is being used for a distal rectal perforation, then it is mandatory to lavage the bowel distal to the defunctioning loop colostomy to remove all fecal material. This will make the loop colostomy more efficient in its primary indication to decompress and defunction the distal rectum. Longer-term complications include leakage at the stoma from poor appliance fit.

Major Complications

Failure to function to decompress and defunction the more distal colon may require further surgery. **Stomal ischemia** and **perforation** with **leakage and wound infection** may lead to **abscess formation**, subcutaneously or intraabdominally, sometimes with **peritonitis** and **systemic sepsis**. **Stomal retraction or prolapse** can be major problems requiring revisional surgery. **Multi-system organ failure** may then occur. Local complications such as **fistula formation**, **cellulitis**, and **external leakage** can be a major problem for the patient and staff.

Consent and Risk Reduction

Main Points to Explain

- GA risk
- Wound infection
- Abscess formation
- Bleeding
- Stoma problems
- Possible injury to blood vessels and bowel
- Risks of reversal
- Further surgery

Large Bowel Resection Right Hemicolectomy (Colostomy and Ileostomy Without Anastomosis)

Description

General anesthetic is used. The patient is placed in the supine position, occasionally the modified Lloyd-Davies position may be used if extended right hemicolectomy is performed. A urinary catheter is placed in the bladder. Preoperative sitting, ideally by a stomal therapy nurse, is highly recommended. In an emergency setting, siting the stoma may not be possible, and the aperture of the stoma is best placed in a horizontal plane in the right iliac fossa adjacent to the umbilicus. The stoma should ideally go through the rectus muscle.

Often, the reason for not performing an anastomosis is the presence of intraabdominal sepsis arising from perforation, typically associated with Crohn's disease or other inflammatory processes of the ileocecal region. Occasionally, small bowel obstruction associated with malignant or inflammatory processes of the right colon is a reason for right hemicolectomy. Dilatation of the small bowel often mitigates against a safe anastomosis. In any other circumstances where anastomosis is contraindicated, then an ileostomy should be fashioned.

The objective of this operation is to perform mobilization of the right colon, including the cecum, hepatic flexure, and transverse colon from the omentum with control of the blood supply involving ligation of the ileocolic, right colic, and branches of the middle colic artery; resection of the dissected bowel; and creation of an end ileostomy and mucous fistula of the colon.

If a stoma is being considered, a midline incision is performed. For most other operations involving the right colon, an upper transverse incision affords good access.

It is important to align the fascia/muscle/skin openings so as not to "scissor" the opening which can cause outlet obstruction. Designing the correct sized opening for the bowel caliber is vital to avoid narrowing due to a too small opening or pro-lapse/hernia due to a too large opening. The pathology, degree of bowel edema, and anatomical location (e.g., colon vs. ileum) can influence this at the time of surgery. The authors prefer an end ileostomy with staple closure of the colon. Alternatively, the ileum and colon may be brought out through the same aperture, and the back wall of a tension-free anastomosis created using continuous mono-filament absorbable suture material, a rod placed under the suture line (i.e., FG8 infant feeding tube), and a modified Brooke-type ileostomy fashioned. A Brooke ostomy often improves appliance fitting and thereby decreases skin irritation from the ostomy contents and skin contraction. This will make the second stage of the operation, viz., ileocolonic anastomosis, more straightforward, avoiding a formal laparotomy.

Anatomical Points

The main anatomical variant is malrotation with the cecum in the right upper quad-rant. Rarely, situs inversus may occur with the cecum on the left. Pathology may alter anatomy, reducing mobility and producing indurated tissues, sometimes dictat-ing the surgical options.

Perspective

See Table 2.7. Many of the complications are not particularly severe, and most relate to the stoma itself or sepsis arising from the underlying disease process. Ischemic necrosis of the ileostomy is the most significant problem encountered but often avoided by making an adequate sized aperture of and ensuring arterial blood supply to the ileum and colon before abdominal closure. Longer-term complica-tions include leakage from stoma from poor appliance fit. Although mortality is usually low, in cases with comorbidities, obstructed bowel, or established infection, risk of morbidity and mortality may be significantly increased, and this should be taken into account in these settings.

Table 2.7 Right hemicolectomy (colostomy and ileostomy <u>without</u> primary anastomosis) estimated frequency of complications, risks, and consequences

Complications, risks, and consequences	Estimated frequency
Most significant/serious complications	
Infection[a] overall	5–20 %
Subcutaneous	5–20 %
Intraabdominal/pelvic (peritonitis, abscess)	1–5 %
Systemic sepsis[a]	0.1–1 %
Hepatic portal sepsis (rare)	<0.1 %
Bleeding/hematoma formation[a]	
Wound	1–5 %
Intraabdominal	1–5 %
Electrolyte/fluid disturbance	5–20 %
Retraction of stoma	1–5 %
Stomal prolapse	0.1–1 %
Stomal stenosis/obstruction	0.1–1 %
Parastomal hernia formation	1–5 %
Multi-system failure (renal, pulmonary, cardiac failure)[a]	1–5 %
Death[a]	1–5 %
Rare significant/serious problems	
Small bowel obstruction (early or late)[a]	0.1–1 %
[Anastomotic stenosis/adhesion formation]	
Entero-cutaneous fistula[a]	0.1–1 %
Ischemic bowel necrosis	0.1–1 %
Misorientation[a]	0.1–1 %
Duodenal injury	0.1–1 %
Wound dehiscence	0.1–1 %
Deep venous thrombosis	0.1–1 %
Ureteric injury (v. rare)[a]	<0.1 %
Vascular injury (v. rare)[a]	<0.1 %
Less serious complications	
Paralytic ileus	50–80 %
Seroma formation	0.1–1 %
Stomal ulceration	1–5 %
Stomal leakage (poor sealing of bag)	1–5 %
Malpositioning of colostomy/ileostomy	0.1–1 %
Cutaneous infective sinus (abscess associated)	0.1–1 %
Nutritional deficiency – anemia, B12 malabsorption[a]	0.1–1 %
Incisional hernia (delayed heavy lifting/straining for 8 weeks)	0.1–1 %
Wound scarring (poor cosmesis/wound deformity)[a]	50–80 %
Pain/tenderness [wound pain]	
Acute (<4 weeks)	>80 %
Chronic (>12 weeks)	1–5 %
Nasogastric tube[a]	1–5 %
Wound drain tube(s)[a]	1–5 %

[a]Dependent on underlying pathology, anatomy, situational factors, surgical technique, and preferences

Major Complications

Stomal ischemia and **stomal necrosis** represent a spectrum from chronic minor problems to severe **stomal retraction, leakage, peritonitis, abscess formation,** and **fistula formation. Systemic sepsis** and very rarely **multi-system organ failure** may supervene. **Small bowel obstruction** is an uncommon complication, but can be a severe problem with recurrent episodes and sometimes requiring repeated surgery for division of adhesions. **Ureteric injury** is very rare, but the cecum and ascending colon are anteriorly related to the right ureter. **Further surgery** may be required for correction of any of the above problems or for later ileocolic anastomosis to restore bowel continuity.

Consent and Risk Reduction

Main Points to Explain

- GA risk
- Wound infection
- Abscess formation
- Bleeding
- Stoma problems
- Risks of reversal
- Possible injury to blood vessels, bowel, and ureter
- Further surgery

Right Hemicolectomy (with Primary Ileocolonic Anastomosis)

Description

General anesthetic is used. The patient is placed in the supine position, occasionally the modified Lloyd-Davies position may be used if extended right hemicolectomy is performed. A urinary catheter is placed in the bladder. Either a midline incision or an upper transverse incision may be used.

The objective of this operation is to perform mobilization and resection of the right colon including the cecum, ascending colon, hepatic flexure, and proximal transverse colon with ligation of the blood supply particularly the ileocolic, right colic, and branches of the middle colic with primary anastomosis of the ileum to the transverse colon. Occasionally, this is modified to an ileo-cecectomy (limited right hemicolectomy) with an anastomosis of the ileum to the ascending colon, for example, in patients with complicated Crohn's disease, cecal inflammation from appendicitis, or solitary cecal diverticulum. For malignant tumors in the right colon, a right hemicolectomy as described above is preferred. Total mesocolic resection is now advocated for colon cancer.

After ensuring adequate arterial blood supply to both cut ends, particularly the colonic end, the anastomosis may be fashioned either with a continuous single-layer suture technique using absorbable monofilament material with the anastomosis marked with nonabsorbable monofilament suture and Weck clips or with functional end-to-end (or side-to-side) anastomosis using the GIA linear stapler.

Anatomical Points

The main anatomical variant is malrotation with the cecum in the right upper quadrant. Occasionally, situs inversus may occur with the cecum on the left. Pathology may alter anatomy, reducing mobility and producing indurated tissues, sometimes dictating the surgical options.

Perspective

See Table 2.8. Many of the complications are not particularly severe. Anastomotic breakdown is the most serious complication, potentially avoided by not making an anastomosis if the patient's condition mitigates against this, ensuring adequate arterial blood supply at both ends of the bowel and avoidance of tension or twisting of the bowel.

Typically, the small bowel diameter is less than that of the large bowel. A longitudinal (Cheatle) slit incising along the anti-mesenteric border of the small bowel can correct the size disparity. For the stapling technique, the bowel ends are stapled at resection and a side-to-side anastomosis is performed, avoiding the problem of incompatibility of the different diameters of the bowel. Although mortality is usually low, in cases with comorbidities, obstructed bowel, or established infection, risk of morbidity and mortality may be significantly increased, and this should be taken into account in these settings.

Major Complications

Anastomotic breakdown with **leakage** is a serious complication which may result in **local sepsis**, including **abscess formation**, or **generalized peritonitis**. The drainage of an abscess to skin or bowel can result in chronic **sinus** or **fistula** formation. Early or late **small bowel obstruction** may result from either early anastomotic blockage (edema, stenosis, suture misplacement) or from later adhesion formation, which can be a severe problem with recurrent episodes and sometimes requiring

Table 2.8 Right hemicolectomy (with primary ileocolonic anastomosis) estimated frequency of complications, risks, and consequences

Complications, risks, and consequences	Estimated frequency
Most significant/serious complications	
Infection[a] overall	5–20 %
Subcutaneous	5–20 %
Intraabdominal/pelvic (peritonitis, abscess)	1–5 %
Systemic sepsis[a]	0.1–1 %
Hepatic portal sepsis (rare)	<0.1 %
Bleeding/hematoma formation[a]	
Wound	1–5 %
Intraabdominal	1–5 %
Anastomotic breakdown – overall	1–5 %
Fistula formation/abscess/peritonitis	
Stenosis (anastomotic)	0.1–1 %
Diarrhea – bile salt, pseudomembranous, colitis osmotic	
Short term (<4 weeks)	50–80 %
Long term (>12 weeks)	1–5 %
Multi-system failure (renal, pulmonary, cardiac failure)[a]	1–5 %
Death[a]	1–5 %
Rare significant/serious problems	
Small bowel obstruction (early or late)[a]	0.1–1 %
[Anastomotic stenosis/adhesion formation]	
Misorientation[a]	0.1–1 %
Entero-cutaneous fistula	0.1–1 %
Fecal fistula[a]	0.1–1 %
Ischemic bowel necrosis	0.1–1 %
Duodenal injury	0.1–1 %
Wound dehiscence	0.1–1 %
Deep venous thrombosis	0.1–1 %
Ureteric injury (v. rare)[a]	<0.1 %
Vascular injury (v. rare)[a]	<0.1 %
Less serious complications	
Paralytic ileus	50–80 %
Cutaneous infective sinus (abscess associated)	0.1–1 %
Incisional hernia (delayed heavy lifting/straining for 8 weeks)	0.1–1 %
Nutritional deficiency – anemia, B12 malabsorption[a]	0.1–1 %
Wound scarring (poor cosmesis/wound deformity)[a]	50–80 %
Pain/tenderness [wound pain]	
Acute (<4 weeks)	>80 %
Chronic (>12 weeks)	1–5 %
Nasogastric tube[a]	1–5 %
Wound drain tube(s)[a]	1–5 %

[a]Dependent on underlying pathology, anatomy, surgical technique, and preferences

repeated surgery for division of adhesions. **Twisting of the bowel** during anastomotic formation and **injury to other organs** are technical complications, which can occur but are usually rare. **Systemic sepsis** and very rarely **multi-system organ**

failure may supervene. **Ureteric injury** is very rare, but the cecum and ascending colon are anteriorly related to the right ureter. **Further surgery** may be required for correction of any of the above problems.

Consent and Risk Reduction

Main Points to Explain

- GA risk
- Wound infection
- Abscess formation
- Bleeding
- Anastomotic leakage
- Risk of stoma
- Possible injury to blood vessels, bowel, and ureter
- Further surgery

Elective Hartmann's Procedure

Description

General anesthesia is used. Patient is positioned with the urinary catheter in the bladder either in supine or in the modified Lloyd-Davies position. Positioning of the buttocks on the table is important to gain adequate access to the rectum for rectal washout, if necessary. A stomal therapist should preferably be involved in counselling and stomal siting of the patient preoperatively. In the semi-elective setting, this may not be practicable. The ideal site for left iliac fossa colostomy is in horizontal plane 3–4 cm lateral to the umbilicus.

The objective is to resect the (upper) rectosigmoid and close the distal rectal stump and create an end colostomy of the left colon. Elective Hartmann's procedure is performed in those patients where anastomosis is at high risk of failure, usually in the presence of intraabdominal sepsis or unresectable rectal malignancy, or in a patient with medical comorbidities or medical treatment that mitigates against adequate wound healing. The rectum is usually closed with a linear stapler, and it is vital that a supple part of the rectum with adequate blood supply is chosen to avoid breakdown of the staple closure. It is vital to identify and protect the left ureter from injury during rectosigmoid mobilization, particularly when performing transection of the rectum. Preoperative bowel preparation may be useful, but is often not required.

A midline incision is used. Resection of the sigmoid colonic diverticular disease/tumor is usual. Adequate length of the left colon must be achieved before creating a stoma, which will usually involve mobilization of the splenic flexure. The aperture should be wide enough to allow the easy passage of the proximal colon and mesentery through the rectus muscle and abdominal wall. It may be necessary to use a transverse colon for such a stoma. It is important to align the fascia/muscle/skin openings so as not to "scissor" the opening which can cause outlet obstruction. Designing the correct sized opening for the bowel caliber is vital to avoid narrowing due to a too small opening or prolapse/hernia due to a too large opening. The pathology, degree of bowel edema, and anatomical location (e.g., colon vs. ileum) can influence this at the time of surgery.

The abdominal wound is closed with the dressing applied before the colostomy is matured. It is popular to close the proximal colon first with a linear cutter (GIA) to reduce contamination. The problem with this technique is that one cannot be sure that there is arterial blood supply to the cut end of the colon before abdominal closure. It is therefore mandatory to mobilize adequate colon so that a significant length of 5–10 cm can be brought out through the aperture before abdominal closure to avoid tension.

Anatomical Points

The main anatomical variant is malrotation with the colon. Rarely, situs inversus may occur with the descending colon on the right. Pathology may alter anatomy, reducing mobility and producing indurated tissues, sometimes dictating the surgical options. The left ureter may be injured and it is vital to identify and preserve this during mobilization in rectosigmoid surgery.

Perspective

See Table 2.9. Most of the complications are not particularly severe, and most relate to the stoma itself or sepsis arising from the underlying disease process. Ischemic necrosis of the stoma is the major complication to avoid, and this is avoided by taking extra time to perform adequate mobilization of the left colon, by making an adequate sized abdominal wall aperture, and by ensuring adequate blood supply before abdominal closure. Mucocutaneous separation, retraction, and the later complications of colostomy prolapse and peristomal hernia are relatively common. Almost all left iliac fossa colostomies are associated with some form of complication. Involvement of a qualified stomal therapist is mandatory in patient education and follow-up. Septic complications can occasionally be severe and life-threatening. Longer-term complications include leakage from stoma from poor appliance fit.

Table 2.9 Elective Hartmann's procedure estimated frequency of complications, risks, and consequences

Complications, risks, and consequences	Estimated frequency
Most significant/serious complications	
Infection[a] overall	20–50 %
Subcutaneous	5–20 %
Intraabdominal/pelvic (peritonitis, abscess)	5–20 %
Systemic sepsis[a]	5–20 %
Hepatic portal sepsis (rare)	0.1–1 %
Bleeding/hematoma formation[a]	
Wound	1–5 %
Intraabdominal	1–5 %
Electrolyte/fluid disturbance	5–20 %
Retraction of stoma	1–5 %
Stomal prolapse	0.1–1 %
Stomal stenosis/obstruction	0.1–1 %
Parastomal hernia formation	1–5 %
Multi-system failure (renal, pulmonary, cardiac failure)[a]	1–5 %
Death[a]	1–5 %
Rare significant/serious problems	
Rectal stump breakdown/abscess formation	5–20 %
Small bowel obstruction (early or late)[a]	0.1–1 %
[Anastomotic stenosis/adhesion formation]	
Misorientation[a]	0.1–1 %
Entero-cutaneous fistula[a]	0.1–1 %
Ischemic bowel necrosis	0.1–1 %
Duodenal injury	0.1–1 %
Wound dehiscence	0.1–1 %
Deep venous thrombosis	0.1–1 %
Ureteric injury (v. rare)[a]	<0.1 %
Vascular injury (v. rare)[a]	<0.1 %
Less serious complications	
Paralytic ileus	50–80 %
Seroma formation	0.1–1 %
Malpositioning of colostomy	0.1–1 %
Stomal ulceration	1–5 %
Stomal leakage (poor sealing of bag)	1–5 %
Incisional hernia (delayed heavy lifting/straining for 8 weeks)	0.1–1 %
Cutaneous infective sinus (abscess associated)	0.1–1 %
Wound scarring (poor cosmesis/wound deformity)[a]	50–80 %
Pain/tenderness [wound pain]	
Acute (<4 weeks)	>80 %
Chronic (>12 weeks)	1–5 %
Urinary retention[a]	1–5 %
Nasogastric tube[a]	1–5 %
Wound drain tube(s)[a]	1–5 %

[a]Dependent on underlying pathology, anatomy, surgical technique, and preferences

Major Complications

Stomal ischemia and **stomal necrosis** represent a spectrum from chronic minor problems to severe **stomal retraction, leakage, peritonitis, abscess formation,** and **fistula formation**; **systemic sepsis** and very rarely **multi-system organ failure** may supervene. **Small bowel obstruction** is an uncommon complication, but can be a severe problem with recurrent episodes and sometimes requiring repeated surgery for division of adhesions. **Ureteric injury** is very rare, but the rectum and sigmoid colon mesentery are closely related to the left ureter. **Further surgery** may be required for correction of any of the above problems or for later colorectal anastomosis to restore bowel continuity if this is desired.

Consent and Risk Reduction

Main Points to Explain

- GA risk
- Wound infection
- Abscess formation
- Severe sepsis
- Bleeding
- Stoma problems
- Risks of reversal
- Possible injury to blood vessels, bowel, and ureter
- Further surgery

Emergency Hartmann's Procedure

Description

General anesthesia is used. Patient is positioned with the urinary catheter in the bladder either in supine or in the modified Lloyd-Davies position. Positioning of the buttocks on the table is important to gain adequate access to the rectum for rectal washout, if necessary. Preoperative bowel preparation is not usually possible. Because this is a nonelective procedure, a stomal therapist may not be involved in counselling and siting the patient preoperatively. The ideal site for left iliac fossa colostomy is in horizontal plane 3–4 cm lateral to the umbilicus.

The objective is to resect the (upper) rectosigmoid and close the distal rectal stump and create an end colostomy of the left colon. Emergency Hartmann's procedure is performed in those patients where anastomosis is at high risk of failure, usually in the presence of intraabdominal sepsis or unresectable rectal malignancy, or in a patient with medical comorbidities or medical treatment that mitigates against adequate wound healing. In the emergency setting, the additional objective is resection of the perforation site, diseased bowel, and obstructing lesion; debridement of any necrotic tissue; and copious lavage of the peritoneal cavity. The rectum is usually closed with a linear stapler, and it is vital that a supple part of the rectum with adequate blood supply is chosen to avoid breakdown of the staple closure. It is vital to identify and protect the left ureter to avoid injury during rectosigmoid mobilization, particularly when performing transection of the rectum.

A midline incision is used. Adequate length of the left colon must be achieved before creating a stoma. Resection of the sigmoid colonic disease is advisable and this will usually involve mobilization of the splenic flexure. The aperture should be wide enough to allow the passage of the proximal colon and mesentery, and it may be necessary to use a transverse colon for such a stoma. The stoma should ideally go through the rectus muscle.

The abdominal wound is closed with the dressing applied before the colostomy is matured. It is popular to close the proximal colon with a linear cutter (GIA) to reduce contamination. The problem with this technique is that one cannot be sure that there is arterial blood supply to the cut end of the colon before abdominal closure. It may be necessary to use a transverse colon for such a stoma. It is important to align the fascia/muscle/skin openings so as not to "scissor" the opening which can cause outlet obstruction. Designing the correct sized opening for the bowel caliber is vital to avoid narrowing due to a too small opening or prolapse/hernia due to a too large opening. The pathology, degree of bowel edema, and anatomical location (e.g., colon vs. ileum) can influence this at the time of surgery. It is therefore mandatory to mobilize adequate colon so that a significant length of 5–10 cm can be brought out through the aperture before abdominal closure to avoid tension. If fecal contamination is significant, it may be best not to attempt any form of abdominal closure, but leave the abdominal cavity completely open as a laparostomy or occasionally place mesh to achieve abdominal closure (although perhaps associated with a greater chance of small bowel entero-cutaneous fistula). If possible the abdominal wall should be closed, but the skin may be left open with antiseptic gauze applied for later delayed primary closure.

Anatomical Points

The main anatomical variant is malrotation with the colon. Rarely, situs inversus may occur with the descending colon on the right. Pathology may alter anatomy, reducing mobility and producing indurated tissues, sometimes dictating the surgical options. The left ureter may be injured and it is vital to identify and preserve this during mobilization in rectosigmoid surgery.

Perspective

See Table 2.10. Complications are very similar to elective Hartmann's procedure though septic complications are more common. Most of the complications are not particularly severe, and most relate to the stoma itself or sepsis arising from the underlying disease process. Ischemic necrosis of the stoma is the major complication to avoid, and this is avoided by taking extra time to perform adequate mobilization of the left colon, by making an adequate sized abdominal wall aperture, and by ensuring adequate blood supply before abdominal closure. Mucocutaneous separation, retraction, and the later complications of colostomy prolapse and peristomal hernia are relatively common. Almost all left iliac fossa colostomies are associated with some form of complication. Involvement of a qualified stomal therapist is mandatory in patient education and follow-up. Septic complications can occasionally be severe and life-threatening.

Major Complications

Stomal ischemia and **stomal necrosis** represent a spectrum from chronic minor problems to severe **stomal retraction, leakage, peritonitis, abscess formation**, and **fistula formation; systemic sepsis** and very rarely **multi-system organ failure** may supervene. **Small bowel obstruction** is an uncommon complication, but can be a severe problem with current episodes and sometimes requiring repeated surgery for division of adhesions. **Ureteric injury** is very rare, but the rectum and sigmoid colon mesentery are closely related to the left ureter, as may the inflammatory, malignant, or other mass. The right ureter is less likely to be injured but can be with extensive emergency surgery. **Further surgery** may be required for correction of any of the above problems or for later colorectal anastomosis to restore bowel continuity, if desired. Longer-term complications include leakage from stoma from poor appliance fit.

Consent and Risk Reduction

Main Points to Explain

- GA risk
- Wound infection
- Abscess formation
- Bleeding
- Stoma problems
- Risks of reversal
- Possible injury to blood vessels, bowel, and ureter
- Further surgery

Table 2.10 Emergency Hartmann's procedure estimated frequency of complications, risks, and consequences

Complications, risks, and consequences	Estimated frequency
Most significant/serious complications	
Infection[a] overall	50–80 %
Subcutaneous	20–50 %
Intraabdominal/pelvic (peritonitis, abscess)	20–50 %
Systemic sepsis[a]	20–50 %
Hepatic portal sepsis (rare)	1–5 %
Bleeding/hematoma formation[a]	
Wound	1–5 %
Intraabdominal	5–20 %
Electrolyte/fluid disturbance[a]	5–20 %
Rectal stump breakdown/abscess formation	5–20 %
Stomal leakage (poor sealing of bag)	1–5 %
Retraction of stoma	1–5 %
Stomal prolapse	0.1–1 %
Stomal stenosis/obstruction	0.1–1 %
Parastomal hernia formation	1–5 %
Multi-system failure (renal, pulmonary, cardiac failure)[a]	5–20 %
Death[a]	5–20 %
Rare significant/serious problems	
Small bowel obstruction (early or late)[a] [Anastomotic stenosis/adhesion formation]	0.1–1 %
Misorientation[a]	0.1–1 %
Entero-cutaneous fistula[a]	0.1–1 %
Ischemic bowel necrosis	0.1–1 %
Wound dehiscence	0.1–1 %
Deep venous thrombosis	0.1–1 %
Ureteric injury (v. rare)[a]	<0.1 %
Vascular injury (v. rare)[a]	<0.1 %
Less serious complications	
Paralytic ileus	>80 %
Stomal ulceration	1–5 %
Cutaneous infective sinus (abscess associated)	0.1–1 %
Seroma formation	0.1–1 %
Malpositioning of colostomy	0.1–1 %
Incisional hernia (delayed heavy lifting/straining for 8 weeks)	1–5 %
Wound scarring (poor cosmesis/wound deformity)[a]	50–80 %
Pain/tenderness [wound pain]	
Acute (<4 weeks)	>80 %
Chronic (>12 weeks)	1–5 %
Urinary retention[a]	1–5 %
Nasogastric tube[a]	1–5 %
Wound drain tube(s)[a]	1–5 %

[a]Dependent on underlying pathology, anatomy, surgical technique, and preferences

Segmental Colonic Resection (Colostomy <u>Without</u> Primary Anastomosis)

Description

General anesthesia is used. Patient is positioned usually with the urinary catheter in the bladder, either in supine or in the modified Lloyd-Davies position. Positioning of the buttocks on the table is important to gain adequate access to the rectum for rectal washout, if necessary.

This procedure is performed often in the context where it is unsafe to perform a colonic anastomosis because of the presence of intraabdominal sepsis or large bowel obstruction, and in a patient with medical comorbidities or with other risk factors that reduce wound healing capacity, e.g., diabetes, large-dose steroids or immunosuppression, renal failure, or malnutrition. The aim therefore is to resect the diseased bowel, create a stoma using the proximal end, and create a mucous fistula of the distal end. This procedure is often performed in the emergency setting. Preoperative bowel preparation may be useful, where feasible.

A midline incision is usually used. Ideally, the patient should be sited for a stoma preoperatively, but this often is not considered in the emergency setting. The site of a stoma is vital for the success in postoperative stoma therapy, being best placed in the horizontal plane 3–4 cm to the lateral side of the umbilicus, preferably through the rectus muscle. It is important to align the fascia/muscle/skin openings so as not to "scissor" the opening which can cause outlet obstruction. Designing the correct sized opening for the bowel caliber is vital to avoid narrowing due to a too small opening or prolapse/hernia due to a too large opening. The side of the stoma will depend on the location and amount of bowel removed. The pathology, degree of bowel edema, and anatomical location (e.g., colon vs. ileum) can influence this at the time of surgery. The aperture in the skin and the abdominal wall should be adequate so that the proximal large bowel (and the distal large bowel, if desired) can easily be passed through the same or separate aperture(s) with their associated mesenteries. The length of the proximal and distal bowel should be documented using a sterile ruler and a diagram, providing this information clearly written in the operation notes. The main abdominal wound should typically be closed including the abdominal wall, skin, and dressing before any attempt is made to mature the stoma. It has become fashionable to divide the ends of the colon using GIA linear cutter to temporarily close and prevent contamination in the abdominal closure.

Anatomical Points

The main anatomical variant is malrotation with the colon. Rarely, situs inversus may occur with the descending colon on the right. Pathology may alter anatomy, reducing mobility and producing indurated tissues, sometimes dictating the surgical options. The left ureter may be injured and it is vital to identify and preserve this during mobilization in colorectal surgery.

Perspective

See Table 2.11. Most of the complications are not particularly severe, and most relate to the stoma itself or sepsis arising from the underlying disease process. Ischemic necrosis of the stoma is the major complication to avoid, and this is avoided by taking extra time to perform adequate mobilization of the left colon, by making an adequate sized abdominal wall aperture, and by ensuring adequate blood supply before abdominal closure. Mucocutaneous separation, retraction, and the later complications of colostomy prolapse, peristomal hernia, and stenosis are relatively common. Fistula formation from the colon proximal to the stoma can lead to leakage into the subcutaneous tissue and create a peristomal abscess. Involvement of a qualified stomal therapist is mandatory in patient education and follow-up. Septic complications can occasionally be severe and life-threatening. Almost all stomas formed have some form of complication. Longer-term complications include leakage from stoma from poor appliance fit.

Major Complications

Stomal ischemia and **stomal necrosis** represent a spectrum from chronic minor problems to severe **stomal retraction**, **leakage**, **peritonitis**, **abscess formation**, and **fistula formation**; **systemic sepsis** and very rarely **multi-system organ failure** may supervene. **Mortality** is rare and related to severe sepsis, organ failure, and comorbidities. **Small bowel obstruction** is an uncommon complication, but can be a severe problem with recurrent episodes and sometimes requiring repeated surgery for division of adhesions. **Ureteric injury** is very rare, but medial aspect of the colon mesentery is closely related to the left ureter. **Further surgery** may be required for correction of any of the above problems or for later colonic anastomosis to restore bowel continuity.

Consent and Risk Reduction

Main Points to Explain

- GA risk
- Wound infection
- Abscess formation
- Bleeding

- Stoma problems
- Risks of reversal
- Possible injury to blood vessels, bowel, and ureter
- Further surgery

Table 2.11 Segmental colonic resection (colostomy <u>without</u> primary anastomosis) estimated frequency of complications, risks, and consequences

Complications, risks, and consequences	Estimated frequency
Most significant/serious complications	
Infection[a] overall	1–5 %
Subcutaneous	1–5 %
Intraabdominal/pelvic (peritonitis, abscess)	1–5 %
Systemic sepsis[a]	1–5 %
Hepatic portal sepsis (rare)	0.1–1 %
Bleeding[a]	
Wound	1–5 %
Intraabdominal	1–5 %
Hematoma formation	1–5 %
Electrolyte/fluid disturbance	5–20 %
Rectal/colonic stump breakdown/abscess formation	1–5 %
Retraction of stoma	1–5 %
Parastomal hernia formation	1–5 %
Multi-system failure (renal, pulmonary, cardiac failure)[a]	1–5 %
Death	1–5 %
Rare significant/serious problems	
Stomal prolapse	0.1–1 %
Stomal stenosis/obstruction	0.1–1 %
Small bowel obstruction (early or late)[a]	0.1–1 %
[Anastomotic stenosis/adhesion formation]	
Misorientation[a]	0.1–1 %
Entero-cutaneous fistula[a]	0.1–1 %
Ischemic bowel necrosis	0.1–1 %
Splenic injury[a]	0.1–1 %
Conservation (consequent limitation to activity, late rupture)	
Splenectomy	
Duodenal injury[a]	0.1–1 %
Wound dehiscence	0.1–1 %
Deep venous thrombosis	0.1–1 %
Ureteric injury (v. rare)[a]	<0.1 %
Vascular injury (v. rare)[a]	<0.1 %
Less serious complications	
Paralytic ileus	50–80 %
Seroma formation	0.1–1 %
Stomal ulceration	1–5 %
Stomal leakage (poor sealing of bag)	1–5 %

(continued)

Table 2.11 (continued)

Complications, risks, and consequences	Estimated frequency
Cutaneous infective sinus (abscess associated)	0.1–1 %
Diarrhea – bile salt, pseudomembranous colitis, osmotic	
Short term (<4 weeks)	20–50 %
Long term (>12 weeks)	1–5 %
Malpositioning of colostomy	0.1–1 %
Incisional hernia (delayed heavy lifting/straining for 8 weeks)	0.1–1 %
Wound scarring (poor cosmesis/wound deformity)[a]	50–80 %
Pain/tenderness [wound pain]	
Acute (<4 weeks)	>80 %
Chronic (>12 weeks)	1–5 %
Urinary retention[a]	1–5 %
Nasogastric tube[a]	1–5 %
Wound Drain Tube(s)[a]	1–5 %

[a]Dependent on underlying pathology, anatomy, surgical technique, and preferences

Segmental Colonic Resection (with Primary Colonic Anastomosis)

Description

General anesthesia is used. The patient is usually positioned either in the supine or in the modified Lloyd-Davies position to gain adequate access to the rectum and anus and also provide the surgeon with access to mobilize the splenic flexure. A long midline incision is used.

The objective of the operation is to resect the affected colon segment and perform an anastomosis between the proximal colon and the sigmoid colon or the left colon and the rectum. Two most common operations here are left hemicolectomy and sigmoid colectomy. In all operations involving the left colon, mobilization of the splenic flexure is mandatory. The midline abdominal incision therefore needs to be extended well above the umbilicus. After mobilization of the left colon and sigmoid colon on the left, the gonadal vessels and left ureter are identified and preserved. The arterial blood supply to the colon is ligated, and before performing end-to-end anastomosis, it is vital that both ends of the bowel are not under tension and the bowel wall is supple with arterial blood supply present at both ends. Anastomosis may be fashioned either with single-layer continuous suture using a monofilament absorbable material or with a staple technique of many types. The most significant factor in obtaining successful anastomosis is ensuring adequate arterial blood supply, being aware of the anatomy and anatomical points of blood supply, particularly in the two watershed areas at the rectosigmoid junction and the splenic flexure.

Anatomical Points

The main anatomical variant is malrotation with the colon. Rarely, situs inversus may occur with the descending colon on the right. Pathology may alter anatomy, reducing mobility and producing indurated tissues, sometimes dictating the surgical options. The left ureter may be injured and it is vital to identify and preserve this during mobilization in colorectal surgery.

Perspective

See Table 2.12. Many of the complications are not particularly severe. Anastomotic breakdown is the most serious complication, potentially avoided by not making an anastomosis if the patient's condition mitigates against this, ensuring adequate arterial blood supply at both ends of the bowel and avoidance of tension or twisting of the bowel. The diameters of the large bowel may not be equal, and angulation of one side or side-to-side technique may be required to correct the disparity. For the stapling technique, the bowel ends are stapled at resection and a side-to-side anastomosis is performed, avoiding the problem of incompatibility of the different diameters of the bowel.

Major Complications

Anastomotic breakdown with **leakage** is a serious complication which may result in **local sepsis**, including **abscess formation**, or **generalized peritonitis**. The drainage of an abscess to skin or bowel can result in chronic **sinus** or **fistula** formation. Early or late **small bowel obstruction** may result either from early anastomotic blockage (edema, stenosis, suture misplacement) or from later adhesion formation, which can be a severe problem with recurrent episodes and sometimes requiring repeated surgery for division of adhesions. **Twisting of the bowel** during anastomotic formation and **injury to other organs** are technical complications, which can occur but are usually rare. **Systemic sepsis** and very rarely **multi-system organ failure** may supervene. These are the main causes of **mortality** when it occurs. **Ureteric injury** is very rare, but the cecum and ascending colon are closely related to the right ureter, and the left ureter lies at the root of the sigmoid mesentery. When used, diverting **ileal loop stomal** complications can be problematic, including retraction, stenosis, parastomal hernia, ulceration, and local sepsis. **Further surgery** may be required for correction of any of the above problems.

Table 2.12 Segmental colonic resection (with primary colonic anastomosis) estimated frequency of complications, risks, and consequences

Complications, risks, and consequences	Estimated frequency
Most significant/serious complications	
Infection[a] overall	1–5 %
Subcutaneous	1–5 %
Intraabdominal/pelvic (peritonitis, abscess)	1–5 %
Systemic sepsis[a]	0.1–1 %
Hepatic portal sepsis (rare)	<0.1 %
Bleeding/hematoma formation[a]	
Wound	1–5 %
Intraabdominal	1–5 %
Anastomotic breakdown – overall	1–5 %
Fistula formation/abscess/peritonitis	
Stenosis (anastomotic)	0.1–1 %
Rare significant/serious problems	
Multi-system failure (renal, pulmonary, cardiac failure)[a]	0.1–1 %
Small bowel obstruction (early or late)[a]	0.1–1 %
Misorientation[a]	0.1–1 %
Entero-cutaneous fistula[a]	0.1–1 %
Ischemic necrosis	0.1–1 %
Splenic injury[a]	0.1–1 %
Conservation (consequent limitation to activity, late rupture)	
Splenectomy	
Duodenal injury[a]	0.1–1 %
Wound dehiscence	0.1–1 %
Deep venous thrombosis	0.1–1 %
Ureteric injury (v. rare)[a]	<0.1 %
Vascular injury (v. rare)[a]	<0.1 %
Death[a]	0.1–1 %
Less serious complications	
Paralytic ileus	50–80 %
Cutaneous infective sinus (abscess associated)	0.1–1 %
Incisional hernia (delayed heavy lifting/straining for 8 weeks)	0.1–1 %
Nutritional deficiency – anemia, B12 malabsorption[a]	0.1–1 %
[Anastomotic stenosis/adhesion formation]	
Diarrhea – bile salt, pseudomembranous colitis, osmotic	
Short term (<4 weeks)	20–50 %
Long term (>12 weeks)	1–5 %
Wound scarring (poor cosmesis/wound deformity)[a]	50–80 %
Pain/tenderness [wound pain]	
Acute (<4 weeks)	>80 %
Chronic (>12 weeks)	1–5 %
Nasogastric tube[a]	1–5 %
Wound drain tube(s)[a]	1–5 %

[a]Dependent on underlying pathology, anatomy, surgical technique, and preferences

Consent and Risk Reduction

Main Points to Explain

- GA risk
- Wound infection
- Abscess formation
- Bleeding
- Anastomotic leakage
- Risk of stoma
- Possible injury to blood vessels, bowel, and ureter
- Further surgery

Anterior Resection (Rectosigmoidectomy) (with or Without Loop Ileostomy)

This includes four main procedures: **high anterior resection** where anastomosis is greater than 10 cm, **low anterior resection** where the anastomosis lies between 6 and 10 cm, **ultralow anterior resection** where the anastomosis lies within 6 cm from the anal verge, and **colo-anal anastomosis**, with an anastomosis at the dentate line.

Description

General anesthetic is used. The patient is positioned in the modified Lloyd-Davies position for easy access to the anus and low rectum. The patient will usually be seen preoperatively by a stomal therapist and sited either for a left iliac fossa colostomy or for a right iliac fossa ileostomy.

The objective of the operation is to resect the rectosigmoid, usually for cancer. Two widely accepted principles are often employed and debated: high ligation of the interior mesenteric artery and total meso-rectal excision of the rectum outside the fascia propria of the rectum.

The anastomosis is most often achieved using a double stapling technique. Linear staple closure of the mobilized rectum is performed. Anastomosis is fashioned using a circular stapler with the proximal colon. A colonic J-pouch may be fashioned using the proximal colon and a linear cutter (GIA) technique.

Before skin preparation the surgeon should perform rectal examination under anesthesia to assess the level of the pathology with rigid sigmoidoscopy and perform lavage of the rectum with some antiseptic, cytotoxic agent, e.g., betadine or hypochlorite solution. A urinary catheter is placed in the bladder. The services of a urologist may be required if preoperative investigations indicate either the left or the right ureter may be at risk or involved with tumor. The use of double-J stents in the left and right ureter will improve their identification.

A long midline incision is used as mobilization of the splenic flexure is mandatory for adequate length to reach the low pelvis. For colo-anal anastomosis the whole rectum is excised with the aid of a perineal surgeon, and the anastomosis achieved between the colon and the anus at the level of the dentate line. This can sometimes be achieved using a stapling technique but more often requires a suture technique of the colon to the anus. For ultralow anterior resection and colo-anal anastomosis and for some patients having a high anterior resection especially after preoperative chemoradiotherapy, a loop ileostomy is used to defunction the colon and the anastomosis.

The objective of a loop ileostomy is to create a stoma that will defunction a distal anastomosis and reduce the complications of an anastomotic leak. The aperture is made of adequate size in the skin of the abdominal wall to comfortably bring out a loop of distal ileum approximately 40–60 cm from the ileocecal valve not under tension. The proximal and distal ends of the ileum should be marked clearly to ensure the correct fashioning of the spout in the proximal ileum. These procedures are virtually always elective in nature. The aperture of the stoma is best placed in a horizontal plane, along a line from the umbilicus to the anterior superior iliac spine, approximately 3–4 cm lateral to the umbilicus usually on the right side. The stoma should ideally go through the rectus muscle. It is important to align the fascia/muscle/skin openings so as not to "scissor" the opening which can cause outlet obstruction. Designing the correct sized opening for the bowel caliber is vital to avoid narrowing due to a too small opening or prolapse/hernia due to a too large opening.

Anatomical Points

The main anatomical variants are malrotation of the colon and differences in length. Rarely, situs inversus may occur with the descending colon on the right. Pathology may alter anatomy, reducing mobility and producing indurated tissues, sometimes dictating the surgical options. The left ureter may be injured and it is vital to identify and preserve this during mobilization in rectosigmoid surgery.

Perspective

See Table 2.13. Most of the complications are minor, but some can be severe. The relative risks of the procedure increase as the resection and anastomosis approximates the anus. Anastomotic leak and other anastomotic complications of hemorrhage, stenosis, and ischemia leading to lengthy strictures are the most pertinent

Table 2.13 Anterior resection (rectosigmoidectomy) (with or without loop ileostomy) estimated frequency of complications, risks, and consequences

Complications, risks, and consequences	Estimated frequency
Most significant/serious complications	
Infection[a] overall	1–5 %
Subcutaneous	1–5 %
Intraabdominal/pelvic (peritonitis, abscess)	1–5 %
Systemic sepsis[a]	1–5 %
Hepatic portal sepsis (rare)	0.1–1 %
Bleeding/hematoma formation[a]	
Wound	1–5 %
Intraabdominal	1–5 %
Anastomotic breakdown – overall	1–5 %
Fistula formation/abscess/peritonitis	
Possible covering loop ileostomy[a,b] (see ileostomy stoma complications)	1–5 %
Functional failure (urgency, intractable diarrhea, painful defecation, incontinence)	1–5 %
Sexual dysfunction[a]	5–20 %
Pelvic tumor recurrence[a]	1–5 %
Parastomal hernia formation[a,b]	1–5 %
Multi-system failure (renal, pulmonary, cardiac failure)[a]	1–5 %
Rare significant/serious problems	
Stenosis (anastomotic)	0.1–1 %
Small bowel obstruction (early or late)[a]	0.1–1 %
[Anastomotic stenosis/adhesion formation]	
Misorientation[a,b]	0.1–1 %
Entero-cutaneous fistula[a]	0.1–1 %
Ischemic bowel necrosis	0.1–1 %
Splenic injury[a]	0.1–1 %
Conservation (consequent limitation to activity; late rupture)	
Splenectomy	
Rectovaginal fistula[a]	0.1–1 %
Bowel injury	0.1–1 %
Bladder injury (possible recto-vesical fistula)	0.1–1 %
Common peroneal injury (esp with Lloyd-Davies type stirrups)	0.1–1 %
Wound dehiscence	0.1–1 %
Deep venous thrombosis	0.1–1 %
Ureteric injury (rare)[a]	0.1–1 %
Vascular injury (rare)[a]	0.1–1 %
Death[a]	0.1–1 %
Less serious complications	
Paralytic ileus	50–80 %
Cutaneous infective sinus (abscess associated)	0.1–1 %
Diarrhea – bile salt, pseudomembranous colitis, osmotic	
Short term (<4 weeks)	20–50 %
Long term (>12 weeks)	1–5 %
Incisional hernia (delayed heavy lifting/straining for 8 weeks)	0.1–1 %

(continued)

Table 2.13 (continued)

Complications, risks, and consequences	Estimated frequency
Nutritional deficiency – anemia, B12 malabsorption[a,b]	0.1–1 %
Wound scarring (poor cosmesis/wound deformity)[a]	50–80 %
Pain/tenderness [wound pain]	
Acute (<4 weeks)	>80 %
Chronic (>12 weeks)	1–5 %
Urinary retention[a]	20–50 %
Nasogastric tube[a]	1–5 %
Wound drain tube(s)[a]	1–5 %

[a]Dependent on underlying pathology, anatomy, surgical technique, and preferences
[b]If a covering ileostomy is used, then complications of this need inclusion

complications. These problems can be reduced by ensuring adequate arterial blood supply at both sides of the anastomosis, splenic flexure mobilization to ensure that proximal colon is not under tension, and avoiding an anastomosis in a patient who has significant risk factors for poor wound healing, particularly in malnutrition, diabetes, and immunosuppression for whatever reason. The anastomosis is often tested on-table at completion of surgery to identify and correct any leaks. Urological complications, particularly injury to the left ureter and bladder, can be avoided by better identification of the ureter and recognizing the position of the bladder, particularly in reopening previous lower midline incisions in women. A common area to injure the left ureter is during transection of the superior rectal artery superior to the sacral promontory, so that identifying the ureter prior to arterial ligation is a safe strategy. Patients with a very distal anastomosis (low or ultralow) may develop the "low anterior resection syndrome" with clustering of bowel movements, urgency, and fecal incontinence, caused by a reduced capacity of the rectum and sphincter stretching. A colonic J-pouch, 6 cm in length, may reduce this problem. Persistent severe diarrhea can occur and may rarely require defunctioning. When a covering ileostomy is used, then complications related to this require inclusion.

Major Complications

Anastomotic breakdown with **leakage** is a serious complication which may result in **local sepsis**, including **abscess formation**, or even **generalized peritonitis**. The drainage of an abscess to skin, bowel, bladder, or vagina can result in chronic and often debilitating **sinus** or **fistula** formation. Early or late **small bowel obstruction** may result from either early or later adhesion formation, which can be a severe problem with recurrent episodes and sometimes requiring repeated surgery for division of adhesions. **Twisting of the bowel** during anastomotic formation and **injury to other organs** are technical complications, which can occur but are usually rare. **Systemic sepsis** and very rarely **multi-system organ failure** may supervene, which is the major cause of **mortality** when it occurs. **Ureteric injury** is very rare with preoperative stenting. **Urinary dysfunction with bladder atony** can be a significant problem. **Ileal loop stomal** complications can be problematic, including retraction, stenosis, parastomal hernia, ulceration, and local sepsis. **Severe diarrhea** can be intractable and a very debilitating problem on occasions. **Further surgery** may be required for correction of any of the above problems. **Sexual dysfunction** may be a severe and particularly debilitating complication for males, with erectile and ejaculatory dysfunction, often reduced by the meso-rectal excision method.

Consent and Risk Reduction

Main Points to Explain

- GA risk
- Wound infection
- Abscess formation
- Bleeding
- Anastomotic leakage
- Risks of a stoma
- Stoma problems
- Possible injury to blood vessels, bowel, and ureter
- Sexual, bladder, and bowel dysfunction
- Difficult bowel control
- Further surgery

Restoration of Continuity Following Right Hemicolectomy, Hartmann's Procedure, Segmental Colonic Resection, and Low Anterior Resection (Open or Laparoscopic)*

Description

General anesthesia is used. The patient is usually positioned supine. Preoperative colonoscopy may be prudent to exclude recent colorectal pathology, depending on the time since initial surgery. The objective of the operation is to restore continuity to the colon by closing the loop colostomy, rejoining the double-barreled colostomy, or anastomosis of the rectal stump with the mobilized left colon after takedown of the colostomy following a previous Hartmann's procedure. The anastomosis can be achieved by direct end-to-end closure (which may require limited colonic resection) using sutures or a double circular stapling device or occasionally a side-to-side approach using a linear stapler. The degree of dissection, resection, and difficulty is highly variable depending on the initial surgery performed and the presence or absence of scarring and adhesions. Closure of a loop colostomy can vary from a small, localized procedure to a large difficult high-risk procedure within the pelvis. The restoration of continuity procedures is virtually always elective in nature.

Anatomical Points

The main anatomical variants are malrotation of the colon and length differences. Rarely, situs inversus may occur with the descending colon on the right. Pathology may alter anatomy, reducing mobility and producing indurated tissues and scarring, sometimes dictating the surgical options. The ureters may be vulnerable depending on the degree of dissection required and should be identified and preserved.

Perspective

See Table 2.14. Most of the complications are minor, but some can be severe. Anastomotic leak and other anastomotic complications of hemorrhage, stenosis, and ischemia leading to lengthy strictures are the most pertinent complications. These problems can be avoided by ensuring adequate arterial blood supply at both sides of the anastomosis, splenic flexure mobilization to ensure that proximal colon is not under tension, and avoiding an anastomosis in a patient who has significant risk factors for poor wound healing, particularly in malnutrition, diabetes, and immunosuppression for whatever reason. Urological complications, particularly injury to the left ureter and bladder, can be avoided by better identification of the ureter and recognizing the position of the bladder, particularly in reopening previous lower midline incisions in women. Patients with a low distal anastomosis may develop the "anterior resection syndrome" of urgency and fecal incontinence caused by a reduced capacity of the rectum and sphincter stretching. Persistent severe diarrhea can occur and may rarely require defunctioning. Patient's age and comorbidities may dictate the wisdom of reversal or not, as mortality and morbidity have been associated with these factors. Laparoscopic reversal can be used, and risks associated with laparoscopic approaches need consideration.

Major Complications

Anastomotic breakdown with **leakage** is a serious complication which may result in **local sepsis**, including **abscess formation**, or even **generalized peritonitis**. **Systemic sepsis** and very rarely **multi-system organ failure** may supervene, which is the major cause of **mortality** when it occurs. The drainage of an abscess to skin, bowel, bladder, or vagina can result in chronic and often debilitating **sinus** or **fistula** formation. Early or late **small bowel obstruction** may result from either early or later adhesion formation, which can be a severe problem with recurrent episodes and sometimes requiring repeated surgery for division of adhesions. **Twisting of the bowel** during anastomotic

Table 2.14 Restoration of continuity following right hemicolectomy, Hartmann's procedure, segmental colonic resection, low anterior resection (open or laparoscopic) estimated frequency of complications, risks, and consequences

Complications, risks, and consequences	Estimated frequency
Most significant/serious complications	
Infection[a] overall	5–20 %
Subcutaneous	1–5 %
Intraabdominal/pelvic (peritonitis, abscess)	5–20 %
Systemic sepsis[a]	1–5 %
Hepatic portal sepsis (rare)	0.1–1 %
Bleeding/hematoma formation[a]	
Wound	1–5 %
Intraabdominal	1–5 %
Anastomotic breakdown – overall	5–20 %
Fistula formation/abscess/peritonitis	
Anastomotic stenosis	0.1–1 %
Possible covering loop ileostomy[a] (see ileostomy complications)	1–5 %
Functional failure[a] (urgency, intractable diarrhea, painful defecation, incontinence)	1–5 %
Parastomal hernia formation	1–5 %
For difficult pelvic surgery	
Sexual dysfunction[a]	5–20 %
Dysplasia or cancer (subsequently)[a]	1–5 %
Proctitis[a]	1–5 %
Multi-system failure (renal, pulmonary, cardiac failure)[a]	1–5 %
Death[a]	1–5 %
Rare significant/serious problems	
Small bowel obstruction (early or late)[a]	0.1–1 %
[Anastomotic stenosis/adhesion formation]	
Misorientation[a]	0.1–1 %
Entero-cutaneous fistula[a]	0.1–1 %
Ischemic bowel necrosis	0.1–1 %
Splenic injury (direct or traction on adhesions to spleen)[a]	0.1–1 %
Conservation (consequent limitation to activity, late rupture)	
Splenectomy	
Deep venous thrombosis	0.1–1 %
Bowel injury	0.1–1 %
Common peroneal injury (esp with Lloyd-Davies type stirrups)	0.1–1 %
Vascular injury (rare)[a]	0.1–1 %
Wound dehiscence	0.1–1 %
For difficult pelvic surgery	
Rectovaginal fistula (female)	0.1–1 %
Infertility[a] (female – adhesions; loss of tubal patency)	0.1–1 %
Bladder injury (possible recto-vesical fistula)	0.1–1 %
Failure to reach distal bowel limb	0.1–1 %
Ureteric injury (rare)[a]	<0.1 %
Less serious complications	
Paralytic ileus	50–80 %

(continued)

Table 2.14 (continued)

Complications, risks, and consequences	Estimated frequency
Cutaneous infective sinus (abscess associated)	0.1–1 %
Diarrhea – bile salt, pseudomembranous colitis, osmotic	
Short term (<4 weeks)	20–50 %
Long term (>12 weeks)	1–5 %
Incisional hernia (delayed heavy lifting/straining for 8 weeks)	0.1–1 %
Nutritional deficiency – anemia, B12 malabsorption[a]	0.1–1 %
Wound scarring (poor cosmesis/wound deformity)[a]	50–80 %
Pain/tenderness [wound pain]	
Acute (<4 weeks)	>80 %
Chronic (>12 weeks)	1–5 %
Urinary retention/catheterization[a]	20–50 %
Nasogastric tube[a]	1–5 %
Wound drain tube(s)[a]	1–5 %

[a]Dependent on underlying pathology, anatomy, surgical technique, and preferences

formation and **injury to other organs** are technical complications, which can occur but are usually rare. **Ureteric injury** is very rare with preoperative stenting. **Ileal loop stomal** complications can be problematic, including retraction, stenosis, parastomal hernia, ulceration, and local sepsis. **Severe diarrhea** can be intractable and a very debilitating problem on occasions. **Further surgery** may be required for correction of any of the above problems. After rectal mobilization, **sexual dysfunction** may be a severe and particularly debilitating complication for males, with erectile and ejaculatory dysfunction reduced by the meso-rectal excision method.

Consent and Risk Reduction

Main Points to Explain

- GA risk
- Wound infection
- Abscess formation
- Bleeding
- Anastomotic leakage
- Risk of further stoma

Abdominoperineal Resection of the Rectum

Description

General anesthetic is used. The patients will typically be seen preoperatively by a stomal therapist and sited for a left iliac fossa colostomy.

Abdominoperineal excision is often performed with two operating surgeons working, one from above to mobilize the rectum and one below to excise the anus, perineal tissues, and tumor, to meet within the pelvis. The services of a plastic surgeon may also be involved if flap reconstruction of the perineal wound is planned. The procedure is virtually always elective in nature.

The objective of the operation is to resect the anus and rectum, almost always for anal or low rectal cancer, in a situation where a low anastomosis is inappropriate or impossible. The patient is positioned in the modified Lloyd-Davies position for easy access to the abdomen, anus, and low rectum. Before skin preparation the surgeon should perform rectal examination under anesthesia to assess the level of the pathology with rigid sigmoidoscopy and perform lavage of the rectum with some antiseptic, cytotoxic agent, e.g., betadine or hypochlorite solution. A urinary catheter is placed in the bladder. The services of a urologist may be required if preoperative investigations indicate either the left or the right ureter may be at risk or involved with tumor. The use of double-J stents in the left and right ureter will improve their identification.

A long midline incision is used as mobilization of the splenic flexure is mandatory for adequate length to reach the abdominal wall for the colostomy. Two widely accepted principles are often employed and debated: high ligation of the interior mesenteric artery and total meso-rectal excision of the rectum outside the fascia propria of the rectum. Linear staple closure of the mobilized proximal colon is often performed for later fashioning of the stoma. The stoma is best placed in a horizontal plane, approximately 3–4 cm lateral to the umbilicus in the abdominal wall, an end colostomy on the left or an ileostomy on the right, and should ideally go through the rectus muscle. It is important to align the fascia/muscle/skin openings so as not to "scissor" the opening which can cause outlet obstruction. Designing the correct sized opening for the bowel caliber is vital to avoid narrowing due to a too small opening or prolapse/hernia due to a too large opening. A tight stoma can produce venous congestion, edema, and poor wound healing and may lead to retraction and obstruction. Edema usually settles after a few days, as third-space fluid losses redistribute.

The perineal wound is closed by the perineal surgeon with or without a local skin flap reconstruction.

Anatomical Points

The main anatomical variants are malrotation of the colon and differences in length. Rarely, situs inversus may occur with the descending colon on the right. Pathology may alter anatomy, reducing mobility and producing indurated tissues, sometimes dictating the surgical options. The left ureter may be injured and it is vital to identify and preserve this during mobilization in rectosigmoid surgery.

Perspective

See Table 2.15. Most of the complications are not particularly severe, and most relate to the stoma itself or sepsis arising from the underlying disease process.

Some can be severe. Ischemic necrosis of the stoma is a major complication, best avoided by taking extra time to perform adequate mobilization of the left colon, by making an adequate sized abdominal wall aperture, and by ensuring adequate blood supply before abdominal closure. Mucocutaneous separation, retraction, and the later complications of colostomy prolapse, peristomal hernia, and stenosis are collectively common. Fistula formation from the colon proximal to the stoma can lead to small bowel content leaking into the subcutaneous tissue and create a peristomal abscess. Involvement of a qualified stomal therapist is mandatory in patient education and follow-up. Septic complications can occasionally be severe and life-threatening. Almost all stomas formed have some form of complication. Low rectal procedures also carry the risk of sexual dysfunction, particularly in males, and ureteric injury. Urological complications, particularly injury to the left ureter and bladder, can be avoided by better identification of the ureter and recognizing the position of the bladder, particularly in reopening previous lower midline incisions in women. A common area to injure the left ureter is during transection of the superior rectal artery superior to the sacral promontory, so that identifying the ureter prior to arterial ligation is a safe strategy. Abscess and hematoma formation may occur and are often associated with systemic sepsis and chronic perineal, cutaneous, vaginal, and sometimes small bowel fistulae.

Major Complications

Stomal ischemia and **stomal necrosis** represent a spectrum from chronic minor problems to severe **stomal retraction**, **leakage**, **peritonitis**, **abscess formation**, and **fistula formation**; **systemic sepsis** and very rarely **multi-system organ failure** may supervene, which is the major cause of **mortality** when it occurs. The drainage of an abscess to skin, bowel, bladder, or vagina can result in chronic and often debilitating **sinus** or **fistula** formation. **Perineal wound dehiscence** with or without a fistula is not uncommon and will usually heal over months. A **non-healing perineal wound** can occur after or with radiotherapy. **Small bowel obstruction** is an uncommon complication, but can be a severe problem with recurrent episodes and sometimes requiring repeated surgery for division of adhesions. **Ureteric injury** is very rare with preoperative stenting. **Urinary dysfunction with bladder atony** can be a significant problem. **Severe perineal sepsis** and **Fournier's gangrene** are rare but serious problems. **Further surgery** may be required for correction of any of the above problems or for later colonic anastomosis to restore bowel continuity. **Sexual dysfunction** may be a severe and particularly debilitating complication particularly for males, with erectile and ejaculatory dysfunction, reduced by the meso-rectal excision method, depending on the tumor site.

Table 2.15 Abdominoperineal resection of the rectum estimated frequency of complications, risks, and consequences

Complications, risks, and consequences	Estimated frequency
Most significant/serious complications	
Infection[a] overall	1–5 %
Subcutaneous	1–5 %
Intraabdominal/pelvic (peritonitis, abscess)	1–5 %
Systemic sepsis[a]	1–5 %
Hepatic portal sepsis (rare)	0.1–1 %
Fournier's gangrene	<0.1 %
Bleeding/hematoma formation[a]	
Wound	1–5 %
Intraabdominal	1–5 %
Electrolyte/fluid disturbance	5–20 %
Sexual dysfunction[a]	5–20 %
Rectal/colonic stump breakdown/abscess formation	1–5 %
Stomal leakage (poor sealing of bag)	1–5 %
Retraction of stoma	1–5 %
Parastomal hernia formation	1–5 %
Perineal dehiscence/prolapse/herniation/delayed wound healing	1–5 %
Perineal sinus/fistula	1–5 %
Pelvic tumor recurrence[a]	1–5 %
Urethral injury	1–5 %
Urethral stricture	1–5 %
Multi-system failure (renal, pulmonary, cardiac failure)[a]	1–5 %
Death[a]	1–5 %
Rare significant/serious problems	
Stomal prolapse	0.1–1 %
Stomal stenosis/obstruction	0.1–1 %
Parastomal fistula formation	0.1–1 %
Malpositioning of colostomy	0.1–1 %
Ureteric injury (rare)[a]	0.1–1 %
Bladder injury (possible recto-vesical fistula)	0.1–1 %
Small bowel obstruction (early or late)[a]	0.1–1 %
[Anastomotic stenosis/adhesion formation]	
Misorientation[a]	0.1–1 %
Entero-cutaneous fistula[a]	0.1–1 %
Ischemic bowel necrosis	0.1–1 %
Splenic injury[a]	0.1–1 %
Conservation (consequent limitation to activity, late rupture)	
Splenectomy	
Wound dehiscence	0.1–1 %
Perineal tumor recurrence	0.1–1 %
Rectovaginal fistula[a]	0.1–1 %
Deep venous thrombosis	0.1–1 %
Bowel injury	0.1–1 %
Common peroneal injury (esp with Lloyd-Davies type stirrups)	0.1–1 %
Vascular injury (rare)[a]	0.1–1 %

(continued)

Table 2.15 (continued)

Complications, risks, and consequences	Estimated frequency
Less serious complications	
Paralytic ileus	50–80 %
Stomal ulceration	1–5 %
Seroma formation	0.1–1 %
Cutaneous infective sinus (abscess associated)	0.1–1 %
Wound scarring (poor cosmesis/wound deformity)[a]	50–80 %
Pain/tenderness [wound pain]	
Acute (<4 weeks)	>80 %
Chronic (>12 weeks)	1–5 %
Incisional hernia (delayed heavy lifting/straining for 8 weeks)	0.1–1 %
Urinary retention/catheterization[a]	20–50 %
Nasogastric tube[a]	1–5 %
Blood transfusion	0.1–1 %
Wound drain tube(s)[a]	1–5 %

[a]Dependent on underlying pathology, anatomy, surgical technique, and preferences

Consent and Risk Reduction

Main Points to Explain

- GA risk
- Wound infection
- Abscess formation
- Bleeding
- Stoma problems
- Possible injury to blood vessels, bowel, and ureter
- Sexual, bladder, and bowel dysfunction
- Perineal abscess, fistula, and sinus
- Further surgery

Possible Injury to Blood Vessels, Bowel, and Ureter

- Difficult bowel control
- Mortality risk
- Further surgery

Total Procto-colectomy and Restorative Ileo-anal (or Ilio-rectal) Pouch Reconstruction

Description

General anesthetic is used. These procedures are virtually always elective in nature.

Ideally, all patients are counselled preoperatively by a stomal therapist, and sites marked for a loop ileostomy on either side, most commonly on the right.

The objective of the operation is to resect the entire colon and rectum almost to the dentate line, usually for ulcerative colitis, severe polyposis, or cancer. If the rectum is to be resected, then total meso-rectal excision of the rectum outside the fascia propria of the rectum is desirable. The ileum is mobilized down to reach the pelvis, where a "J," "S," "W," or other type of construction can be fashioned. Either a hand-sewn or circular double stapling method can be used.

The patient is positioned in the modified Lloyd-Davies position for easy access to the abdomen, anus, and low rectum. Before skin preparation the surgeon should perform rectal examination under anesthesia to assess the level of the pathology with rigid sigmoidoscopy and perform lavage of the rectum with some antiseptic, cytotoxic agent, e.g., betadine or hypochlorite solution.

A urinary catheter is placed in the bladder. The services of a urologist may be required if preoperative investigations indicate either the left or the right ureter may be at risk or involved with tumor. The use of double-J stents in the left and right ureter will improve their identification. A long midline incision is used as mobilization of the ileum is mandatory for adequate length to reach the low pelvis. A covering ileostomy stoma, when used, is best placed in a horizontal plane, in the right abdominal wall, approximately 3–4 cm lateral to the umbilicus, and should ideally go through the rectus muscle. It is important to align the fascia/muscle/skin openings so as not to "scissor" the opening which can cause outlet obstruction. Designing the correct sized opening for the bowel caliber is vital to avoid narrowing due to a too small opening or prolapse/hernia due to a too large opening. A tight stoma can produce venous congestion, edema, and poor wound healing and may lead to retraction and obstruction. Edema usually settles after a few days, as third-space fluid losses redistribute.

Anatomical Points

The main anatomical variant is malrotation with the colon. Rarely, situs inversus may occur with the descending colon on the right. Pathology may alter anatomy, reducing mobility and producing indurated tissues, sometimes dictating the surgical options. Either ureter may be injured, and it is vital to identify and preserve these during mobilization in colorectal surgery.

Perspective

See Table 2.16. Most of the complications are minor, but some can be severe. Anastomotic leak and other anastomotic complications of hemorrhage, stenosis, and ischemia leading to lengthy strictures are the most pertinent complications.

Table 2.16 Total procto-colectomy and restorative ileo-anal (or ilio-rectal) pouch reconstruction estimated frequency of complications, risks, and consequences

Complications, risks, and consequences	Estimated frequency
Most significant/serious complications	
Infection[a] overall	1–5 %
Subcutaneous	1–5 %
Intraabdominal/pelvic (peritonitis, abscess)	1–5 %
Systemic sepsis[a]	1–5 %
Hepatic portal sepsis (rare)	0.1–1 %
Bleeding/hematoma formation[a]	
Wound	1–5 %
Intraabdominal	1–5 %
Sexual dysfunction[a]	5–20 %
Anastomotic breakdown – overall	1–5 %
Fistula formation/abscess/peritonitis	
Pouch failure or loss	5–10 %
Possible covering loop ileostomy[a] (see ileostomy complications)	20–50 %
Functional failure (urgency, intractable diarrhea, painful defecation, incontinence)	1–5 %
Pelvic tumor recurrence[a]	1–5 %
Parastomal hernia formation	1–5 %
Urethral injury	1–5 %
Urethral stricture	1–5 %
Multi-system failure (renal, pulmonary, cardiac failure)[a]	1–5 %
Death[a]	0.1–1 %
Rare significant/serious problems	
Small bowel obstruction (early or late)[a]	0.1–1 %
[Anastomotic stenosis/adhesion formation]	
Misorientation[a]	0.1–1 %
Stenosis (anastomotic)	0.1–1 %
Entero-cutaneous fistula[a]	0.1–1 %
Ischemic bowel necrosis	0.1–1 %
Pouch-vaginal fistula[a]	0.1–1 %
Bladder (urinary) fistula	0.1–1 %
Infertility (adhesions, loss of tubal patency)	0.1–1 %
Permanent ileostomy	0.1–1 %
Dysplasia or cancer (in residual rectum or pouch)[a]	0.1–1 %
Failure to reach anus	0.1–1 %
Splenic injury[a] (direct or traction on adhesions to spleen)	0.1–1 %
Conservation (consequent limitation to activity, late rupture)	
Splenectomy	
Deep venous thrombosis	0.1–1 %
Bowel injury	0.1–1 %
Bladder injury (possible recto-vesical fistula)	0.1–1 %
Wound dehiscence	0.1–1 %
Deep venous thrombosis	0.1–1 %
Common peroneal injury (esp with Lloyd-Davies type stirrups)	0.1–1 %
Ureteric injury (rare)[a]	0.1–1 %
Vascular injury (rare)[a]	0.1–1 %

Table 2.16 (continued)

Complications, risks, and consequences	Estimated frequency
Less serious complications	
Paralytic ileus	50–80 %
Diarrhea	
Bile salt, pseudomembranous colitis, osmotic	
Overflow (small frequent bowel actions), fecal urgency	
Short term (<4 weeks)	20–50 %
Long term (>12 weeks)	1–5 %
Cutaneous infective sinus (abscess associated)	0.1–1 %
Pouchitis	1–5 %
Incisional hernia (delayed heavy lifting/straining for 8 weeks)	0.1–1 %
Nutritional deficiency – anemia, B12 malabsorption[a]	0.1–1 %
Wound scarring (poor cosmesis/wound deformity)[a]	50–80 %
Pain/tenderness [wound pain]	
Acute (<4 weeks)	>80 %
Chronic (>12 weeks)	1–5 %
Urinary retention[a]	20–50 %
Nasogastric tube/catheterization[a]	1–5 %
Wound drain tube(s)[a]	1–5 %

[a]Dependent on underlying pathology, anatomy, surgical technique, and preferences

These problems can be avoided by ensuring adequate arterial blood supply at both sides of the anastomosis, good ileal mobilization to minimize tension, and avoiding an anastomosis in a patient who has significant risk factors for poor wound healing, particularly in malnutrition, diabetes, and immunosuppression for whatever reason. The anastomosis is often tested on-table at completion of surgery to identify and correct any leaks. Urological complications, particularly injury to the ureters and bladder, can be avoided by identification and recognizing the position of the bladder, particularly in reopening previous lower midline incisions in women. Patients with a very distal anastomosis (low or ultralow) may develop the "low anterior resection syndrome" with clustering of bowel movements, urgency, and fecal incontinence, caused by a reduced capacity of the rectum and sphincter stretching. A colonic J-pouch, 6 cm in length, may reduce this problem. Persistent severe diarrhea can occur and may rarely require defunctioning.

Major Complications

Anastomotic breakdown with **leakage** is a serious complication which may result in **local sepsis,** including **abscess formation,** or even **generalized peritonitis.** **Systemic sepsis** and very rarely **multi-system organ failure** may supervene, which is the major cause of **mortality** when it occurs. The drainage of an abscess to skin, bowel, bladder, or vagina can result in chronic and often debilitating **sinus** or **fistula**

formation. Early or late **small bowel obstruction** may result from either early or later adhesion formation, which can be a severe problem with recurrent episodes and sometimes requiring repeated surgery for division of adhesions. **Twisting of the bowel** during anastomotic formation and **injury to other organs** are technical complications, which can occur, but are usually rare. **Ureteric injury** is very rare with preoperative stenting. **Urinary dysfunction with bladder atony** can be a significant problem. **Ileal loop stomal** complications can be problematic, including retraction, stenosis, parastomal hernia, ulceration, and local sepsis. **Severe diarrhea** can be intractable and a very debilitating problem on occasions. **Further surgery** may be required for correction of any of the above problems. **Sexual dysfunction** may be a severe and particularly debilitating complication for males, with erectile and ejaculatory dysfunction, reduced by the meso-rectal excision method.

Consent and Risk Reduction

Main Points to Explain

- GA risk
- Wound infection
- Abscess formation
- Bleeding
- Anastomotic leakage
- Stoma problems
- Possible injury to blood vessels, bowel, and ureter
- Sexual, bladder, and bowel dysfunction
- Difficult bowel control
- Pouch problems
- Further surgery

Laparoscopic and Robotic-Assisted Laparoscopic (RAL) Colorectal Surgery

Description

All the open operations described above can and are increasingly performed with minimally invasive surgery. The operative techniques follow the principles of minimal invasive surgery, and to describe these in detail is beyond the scope of this book. The complications are similar, however. Minimally invasive surgery has its own complications (e.g., trocar and insufflation related), and these are largely covered in the section on Laparoscopic Appendectomy.

Further Reading, References, and Resources

Rigid Sigmoidoscopy (and/or Rectal Biopsy)

Gatto NM, Frucht H, Sundararajan V, Jacobson JS, Grann VR, Neugut AI. Risk of perforation after colonoscopy and sigmoidoscopy: a population-based study. J Natl Cancer Inst. 2003;95(3): 230–6.

Jamieson GG. The anatomy of general surgical operations. 2nd ed. Edinburgh: Churchill Livingston; 2006.

Colonoscopy

Agalar F, Daphan C, Sayek I, Hayran M. Clinical presentation and management of iatrogenic colon perforations. Am J Surg. 1999;177(5):442.

Ahmed A, Eller PM, Schiffman FJ. Splenic rupture: an unusual complication of colonoscopy. Am J Gastroenterol. 1997;92(7):1201–4. Review.

Anderson ML, Pasha TM, Leighton JA. Endoscopic perforation of the colon: lessons from a 10-year study. Am J Gastroenterol. 2000;95(12):3418–22.

Araghizadeh FY, Timmcke AE, Opelka FG, Hicks TC, Beck DE. Colonoscopic perforations. Dis Colon Rectum. 2001;44(5):713–6.

Basson MD, Etter L, Panzini LA. Rates of colonoscopic perforation in current practice. Gastroenterology. 1998;114(5):1115.

Belo-Oliveira P, Curvo-Semedo L, Rodrigues H, Belo-Soares P, Caseiro-Alves F. Sigmoid colon perforation at CT colonography secondary to a possible obstructive mechanism: report of a case. Dis Colon Rectum. 2007;50(9):1478–80.

Dafnis G, Ekbom A, Pahlman L, Blomqvist P. Complications of diagnostic and therapeutic colonoscopy within a defined population in Sweden. Gastrointest Endosc. 2001;54(3):302–9.

Fletcher RH. Colorectal cancer screening on stronger footing. N Engl J Med. 2008;359:1285–7.

Gatto NM, Frucht H, Sundararajan V, Jacobson JS, Grann VR, Neugut AI. Risk of perforation after colonoscopy and sigmoidoscopy: a population-based study. J Natl Cancer Inst. 2003;95(3): 230–6.

Imperiale TF, Glowinski EA, Lin-Cooper C, Larkin GN, Rogge JD, Ransohoff DF. Five-year risk of colorectal neoplasia after negative screening colonoscopy. N Engl J Med. 2008;359: 1218–24.

Jamieson GG. The anatomy of general surgical operations. 2nd ed. Edinburgh: Churchill Livingston; 2006.

Janes SE, Cowan IA, Dijkstra B. A life threatening complication after colonoscopy. BMJ. 2005;330(7496):88–90. Review.

Korman LY, Overholt BF, Box T, Winker CK. Perforation during colonoscopy in endoscopic ambulatory surgical centers. Gastrointest Endosc. 2003;58(4):554–7.

Levin TR, Zrhao W, Conell C, Seeff LC, Manninen DL, Shapiro JA, Schulman J. Complications of colonoscopy in an integrated health care delivery system. Ann Intern Med. 2006;145(12):880–6. Summary for patients in: Ann Intern Med. 2006;145(12): 139.

Lüning TH, Keemers-Gels ME, Barendregt WB, Tan AC, Rosman C. Colonoscopic perforations: a review of 30,366 patients. Surg Endosc. 2007;21(6):994–7. Review.

Marwan K, Farmer KC, Varley C, Chapple KS. Pneumothorax, pneumomediastinum, pneumoperitoneum, pneumoretroperitoneum and subcutaneous emphysema following diagnostic colonoscopy. Ann R Coll Surg Engl. 2007;89(5):W20–1.

Nelson DB, McQuaid KR, Bond JH, Lieberman DA, Weiss DG, Johnston TK. Procedural success and complications of large-scale screening colonoscopy. Gastrointest Endosc. 2002;55(3): 307–14.

Tiwari A, Melegros L. Colonoscopic perforation. Br J Hosp Med (Lond). 2007;68(8):429–33. Review.

Tran DQ, Rosen L, Kim R, Riether RD, Stasik JJ, Khubchandani IT. Actual colonoscopy: what are the risks of perforation? Am Surg. 2001;67(9):845–7. Discussion 847–8.

Webb T. Pneumothorax and pneumomediastinum during colonoscopy. Anaesth Intensive Care. 1998;26(3):302–4.

Zubarik R, Fleischer DE, Mastropietro C, Lopez J, Carroll J, Benjamin S, Eisen G. Prospective analysis of complications 30 days after outpatient colonoscopy. Gastrointest Endosc. 1999; 50(3):322–8.

Open Appendectomy

Carbonell AM, Burns JM, Lincourt AE, Harold KL. Outcomes of laparoscopic versus open appendectomy. Am Surg. 2004;70(9):759–65. Discussion 765–6.

Cox MR, McCall JL, Toouli J, Padbury RT, Wilson TG, Wattchow DA, Langcake M. Prospective randomized comparison of open versus laparoscopic appendectomy in men. World J Surg. 1996;20(3):263–6.

DesGroseilliers S, Fortin M, Lokanathan R, Khoury N, Mutch D. Laparoscopic appendectomy versus open appendectomy: retrospective assessment of 200 patients. Can J Surg. 1995;38(2):178–82.

Ellis H. Clinical anatomy. 6th ed. Blackwell Scientific Pty Ltd; Oxford, UK 1980.

Frazee RC, Roberts JW, Symmonds RE, Snyder SK, Hendricks JC, Smith RW, Custer 3rd MD, Harrison JB. A prospective randomized trial comparing open versus laparoscopic appendectomy. Ann Surg. 1994;219(6):725–8. Discussion 728–31.

Golub R, Siddiqui F, Pohl D. Laparoscopic versus open appendectomy: a metaanalysis. J Am Coll Surg. 1998;186(5):545–53.

Gupta R, Sample C, Bamehriz F, Birch DW. Infectious complications following laparoscopic appendectomy. Can J Surg. 2006;49(6):397–400.

Hansen JB, Smithers BM, Schache D, Wall DR, Miller BJ, Menzies BL. Laparoscopic versus open appendectomy: prospective randomized trial. World J Surg. 1996;20(1):17–20. Discussion 21.

Hoehne F, Ozaeta M, Sherman B, Miani P, Taylor E. Laparoscopic versus open appendectomy: is the postoperative infectious complication rate different? Am Surg. 2005;71(10):813–5.

Huang MT, Wei PL, Wu CC, Lai IR, Chen RJ, Lee WJ. Needlescopic, laparoscopic, and open appendectomy: a comparative study. Surg Laparosc Endosc Percutan Tech. 2001;11(5):306–12. Erratum in: Surg Laparosc Endosc Percutan Tech. 2002;12(4).

Jamieson GG. The anatomy of general surgical operations. 2nd ed. Edinburgh: Churchill Livingston; 2006.

Kapischke M, Tepel J, Bley K. Laparoscopic appendicectomy is associated with a lower complication rate even during the introductory phase. Langenbecks Arch Surg. 2004;389(6):517–23.

Katkhouda N, Friedlander MH, Grant SW, Achanta KK, Essani R, Paik P, Velmahos G, Campos, G, Mason R, Mavor E. Intraabdominal abscess rate after laparoscopic appendectomy. Am J Surg. 2000;180(6):456–9. Discussion 460–1.

Katkhouda N, Mason RJ, Towfigh S, Gevorgyan A, Essani R. Laparoscopic versus open appendectomy: a prospective randomized double-blind study. Ann Surg. 2005;242(3):439–48. Discussion 448–50.

Kazemier G, de Zeeuw GR, Lange JF, Hop WC, Bonjer HJ. Laparoscopic vs open appendectomy. A randomized clinical trial. Surg Endosc. 1997;11(4):336–40.

Khan MN, Fayyad T, Cecil TD, Moran BJ. Laparoscopic versus open appendectomy: the risk of postoperative infectious complications. JSLS. 2007;11(3):363–7.

Klingler A, Henle KP, Beller S, Rechner J, Zerz A, Wetscher GJ, Szinicz G. Laparoscopic appendectomy does not change the incidence of postoperative infectious complications. Am J Surg. 1998;175(3):232–5.

Kluiber RM, Hartsman B. Laparoscopic appendectomy. A comparison with open appendectomy. Dis Colon Rectum. 1996;39(9):1008–11.

Lin HF, Wu JM, Tseng LM, Chen KH, Huang SH, Lai IR. Laparoscopic versus open appendectomy for perforated appendicitis. J Gastrointest Surg. 2006;10(6):906–10.

Marzouk M, Khater M, Elsadek M, Abdelmoghny A. Laparoscopic versus open appendectomy: a prospective comparative study of 227 patients. Surg Endosc. 2003;17(5):721–4.

McCahill LE, Pellegrini CA, Wiggins T, Helton WS. A clinical outcome and cost analysis of laparoscopic versus open appendectomy. Am J Surg. 1996;171(5):533–7.

McKinlay R, Neeleman S, Klein R, Stevens K, Greenfeld J, Ghory M, Cosentino C. Intraabdominal abscess following open and laparoscopic appendectomy in the pediatric population. Surg Endosc. 2003;17(5):730–3.

Merhoff AM, Merhoff GC, Franklin ME. Laparoscopic versus open appendectomy. Am J Surg. 2000;179(5):375–8.

Minné L, Varner D, Burnell A, Ratzer E, Clark J, Haun W. Laparoscopic vs open appendectomy Prospective randomized study of outcomes. Arch Surg. 1997;132(7):708–11. Discussion 712.

Olmi S, Magnone S, Bertolini A, Croce E. Laparoscopic versus open appendectomy in acute appendicitis: a randomized prospective study. Surg Endosc. 2005;19(9):1193–5.

Ortega AE, Hunter JG, Peters JH, Swanstrom LL, Schirmer B. A prospective, randomized comparison of laparoscopic appendectomy with open appendectomy. Laparoscopic Appendectomy Study Group. Am J Surg. 1995;169(2):208–12. Discussion 212–3.

Sauerland S, Lefering R, Holthausen U, Neugebauer EA. Laparoscopic vs conventional appendectomy–a meta-analysis of randomised controlled trials. Langenbecks Arch Surg. 1998;383(3–4):289–95.

Sauerland S, Lefering R, Neugebauer EA. Laparoscopic versus open surgery for suspected appendicitis. Cochrane Database Syst Rev. 2002;1, CD001546. Review. Update in: Cochrane Database Syst Rev. 2004;(4): CD001546.

Schirmer BD, Schmieg Jr RE, Dix J, Edge SB, Hanks JB. Laparoscopic versus traditional appendectomy for suspected appendicitis. Am J Surg. 1993;165(6):670–5.

Slim K, Pezet D, Chipponi J. Laparoscopic or open appendectomy? Critical review of randomized, controlled trials. Dis Colon Rectum. 1998;41(3):398–403. Review.

Sosa JL, Sleeman D, McKenney MG, Dygert J, Yarish D, Martin L. A comparison of laparoscopic and traditional appendectomy. J Laparoendosc Surg. 1993;3(2):129–31.

Temple LK, Litwin DE, McLeod RS. A meta-analysis of laparoscopic versus open appendectomy in patients suspected of having acute appendicitis. Can J Surg. 1999;42(5):377–83.

Tsao KJ, St Peter SD, Valusek PA, Keckler SJ, Sharp S, Holcomb 3rd GW, Snyder CL, Ostlie DJ. Adhesive small bowel obstruction after appendectomy in children: comparison between the laparoscopic and open approach. J Pediatr Surg. 2007;42(6):939–42. Discussion 942.

Wullstein C, Barkhausen S, Gross E. Results of laparoscopic vs. conventional appendectomy in complicated appendicitis. Dis Colon Rectum. 2001;44(11):1700–5.

Yong JL, Law WL, Lo CY, Lam CM. A comparative study of routine laparoscopic versus open appendectomy. JSLS. 2006;10(2):188–92.

Laparoscopic Appendectomy

Carbonell AM, Burns JM, Lincourt AE, Harold KL. Outcomes of laparoscopic versus open appendectomy. Am Surg. 2004;70(9):759–65. Discussion 765–6.

Cox MR, McCall JL, Toouli J, Padbury RT, Wilson TG, Wattchow DA, Langcake M. Prospective randomized comparison of open versus laparoscopic appendectomy in men. World J Surg. 1996;20(3):263–6.

DesGroseilliers S, Fortin M, Lokanathan R, Khoury N, Mutch D. Laparoscopic appendectomy versus open appendectomy: retrospective assessment of 200 patients. Can J Surg. 1995;38(2):178–82.

Ellis H. Clinical anatomy. 6th ed. Blackwell Scientific Pty Ltd; 1980.

Frazee RC, Roberts JW, Symmonds RE, Snyder SK, Hendricks JC, Smith RW, Custer 3rd MD, Harrison JB. A prospective randomized trial comparing open versus laparoscopic appendectomy. Ann Surg. 1994;219(6):725–8. Discussion 728–31.

Golub R, Siddiqui F, Pohl D. Laparoscopic versus open appendectomy: a metaanalysis. J Am Coll Surg. 1998;186(5):545–53.

Gupta R, Sample C, Bamehriz F, Birch DW. Infectious complications following laparoscopic appendectomy. Can J Surg. 2006;49(6):397–400.

Hansen JB, Smithers BM, Schache D, Wall DR, Miller BJ, Menzies BL. Laparoscopic versus open appendectomy: prospective randomized trial. World J Surg. 1996;20(1):17–20. Discussion 21.

Hoehne F, Ozaeta M, Sherman B, Miani P, Taylor E. Laparoscopic versus open appendectomy: is the postoperative infectious complication rate different? Am Surg. 2005;71(10):813–5.

Huang MT, Wei PL, Wu CC, Lai IR, Chen RJ, Lee WJ. Needlescopic, laparoscopic, and open appendectomy: a comparative study. Surg Laparosc Endosc Percutan Tech. 2001;11(5):306–12. Erratum in: Surg Laparosc Endosc Percutan Tech. 2002;12(4).

Jamieson GG. The anatomy of general surgical operations. 2nd ed. Edinburgh: Churchill Livingston; 2006.

Kapischke M, Tepel J, Bley K. Laparoscopic appendicectomy is associated with a lower complication rate even during the introductory phase. Langenbecks Arch Surg. 2004;389(6):517–23.

Katkhouda N, Friedlander MH, Grant SW, Achanta KK, Essani R, Paik P, Velmahos G, Campos G, Mason R, Mavor E. Intraabdominal abscess rate after laparoscopic appendectomy. Am J Surg. 2000;180(6):456–9. Discussion 460–1.

Katkhouda N, Mason RJ, Towfigh S, Gevorgyan A, Essani R. Laparoscopic versus open appendectomy: a prospective randomized double-blind study. Ann Surg. 2005;242(3):439–48. Discussion 448–50.

Kazemier G, de Zeeuw GR, Lange JF, Hop WC, Bonjer HJ. Laparoscopic vs open appendectomy. A randomized clinical trial. Surg Endosc. 1997;11(4):336–40.

Khan MN, Fayyad T, Cecil TD, Moran BJ. Laparoscopic versus open appendectomy: the risk of postoperative infectious complications. JSLS. 2007;11(3):363–7.

Klingler A, Henle KP, Beller S, Rechner J, Zerz A, Wetscher GJ, Szinicz G. Laparoscopic appendectomy does not change the incidence of postoperative infectious complications. Am J Surg. 1998;175(3):232–5.

Kluiber RM, Hartsman B. Laparoscopic appendectomy: a comparison with open appendectomy. Dis Colon Rectum. 1996;39(9):1008–11.

Lin HF, Wu JM, Tseng LM, Chen KH, Huang SH, Lai IR. Laparoscopic versus open appendectomy for perforated appendicitis. J Gastrointest Surg. 2006;10(6):906–10.

Marzouk M, Khater M, Elsadek M, Abdelmoghny A. Laparoscopic versus open appendectomy: a prospective comparative study of 227 patients. Surg Endosc. 2003;17(5):721–4.

McCahill LE, Pellegrini CA, Wiggins T, Helton WS. A clinical outcome and cost analysis of laparoscopic versus open appendectomy. Am J Surg. 1996;171(5):533–7.

McKinlay R, Neeleman S, Klein R, Stevens K, Greenfeld J, Ghory M, Cosentino C. Intraabdominal abscess following open and laparoscopic appendectomy in the pediatric population. Surg Endosc. 2003;17(5):730–3.

Merhoff AM, Merhoff GC, Franklin ME. Laparoscopic versus open appendectomy. Am J Surg. 2000;179(5):375–8.

Minné L, Varner D, Burnell A, Ratzer E, Clark J, Haun W. Laparoscopic vs open appendectomy. Prospective randomized study of outcomes. Arch Surg. 1997;132(7):708–11. Discussion 712.

Olmi S, Magnone S, Bertolini A, Croce E. Laparoscopic versus open appendectomy in acute appendicitis: a randomized prospective study. Surg Endosc. 2005;19(9):1193–5.

Ortega AE, Hunter JG, Peters JH, Swanstrom LL, Schirmer B. A prospective, randomized comparison of laparoscopic appendectomy with open appendectomy. Laparoscopic Appendectomy Study Group. Am J Surg. 1995;169(2):208–12. Discussion 212–3.

Sauerland S, Lefering R, Holthausen U, Neugebauer EA. Laparoscopic vs conventional appendectomy–a meta-analysis of randomised controlled trials. Langenbecks Arch Surg. 1998; 383(3–4):289–95.

Sauerland S, Lefering R, Neugebauer EA. Laparoscopic versus open surgery for suspected appendicitis. Cochrane Database Syst Rev. 2002;1, CD001546. Review. Update in: Cochrane Database Syst Rev. 2004;(4): CD001546.

Schirmer BD, Schmieg Jr RE, Dix J, Edge SB, Hanks JB. Laparoscopic versus traditional appendectomy for suspected appendicitis. Am J Surg. 1993;165(6):670–5.

Slim K, Pezet D, Chipponi J. Laparoscopic or open appendectomy? Critical review of randomized, controlled trials. Dis Colon Rectum. 1998;41(3):398–403. Review.

Sosa JL, Sleeman D, McKenney MG, Dygert J, Yarish D, Martin L. A comparison of laparoscopic and traditional appendectomy. J Laparoendosc Surg. 1993;3(2):129–31.

Temple LK, Litwin DE, McLeod RS. A meta-analysis of laparoscopic versus open appendectomy in patients suspected of having acute appendicitis. Can J Surg. 1999;42(5):377–83.

Tsao KJ, St Peter SD, Valusek PA, Keckler SJ, Sharp S, Holcomb 3rd GW, Snyder CL, Ostlie DJ. Adhesive small bowel obstruction after appendectomy in children: comparison between the laparoscopic and open approach. J Pediatr Surg. 2007;42(6):939–42. Discussion 942.

Wullstein C, Barkhausen S, Gross E. Results of laparoscopic vs. conventional appendectomy in complicated appendicitis. Dis Colon Rectum. 2001;44(11):1700–5.

Yong JL, Law WL, Lo CY, Lam CM. A comparative study of routine laparoscopic versus open appendectomy. JSLS. 2006;10(2):188–92.

Colostomy and Mucous Fistula

Ansari MZ, Collopy BT, Hart WG, Carson NJ, Chandraraj EJ. In-hospital mortality and associated complications after bowel surgery in Victorian public hospitals. ANZ J Surg. 2000;70(1): 6–10.

Blumetti J, Luu M, Sarosi G, Hartless K, McFarlin J, Parker B, Dineen S, Huerta S, Asolati M, Varela E, Anthony T. Surgical site infections after colorectal surgery: do risk factors vary depending on the type of infection considered? Surgery. 2007;142(5):704–11.

Buchs NC, Gervaz P, Bucher P, Huber O, Mentha G, Morel P. Lessons learned from one thousand consecutive colonic resections in a teaching hospital. Swiss Med Wkly. 2007;137(17–18): 259–64.

Jamieson GG. The anatomy of general surgical operations. 2nd ed. Edinburgh: Churchill Livingston; 2006.

Kim J, Mittal R, Konyalian V, King J, Stamos MJ, Kumar RR. Outcome analysis of patients undergoing colorectal resection for emergent and elective indications. Am Surg. 2007;73(10): 991–3.

Konishi T, Watanabe T, Kishimoto J, Nagawa H. Elective colon and rectal surgery differ in risk factors for wound infection: results of prospective surveillance. Ann Surg. 2006;244(5): 758–63.

Theile DE, Cohen JR, Holt J, Davis NC. Mortality and complications of large-bowel resection for carcinoma. ANZ J Surg. 1979;49(1):62–6.

Loop Colostomy

Bakx R, Busch OR, Bemelman WA, Veldink GJ, Slors J, van Lanschot JJ. Morbidity of temporary loop ileostomies. Dig Surg. 2004;21(4):277–81. 11.

Caricato M, Ausania F, Ripetti V, Bartolozzi F, Campoli G, Coppola R. Retrospective analysis of long-term defunctioning stoma complications after colorectal surgery. Colorectal Dis. 2007;9(6):559–61.

Edwards DP, Leppington-Clarke A, Sexton R, Heald RJ, Moran BJ. Stoma-related complications are more frequent after transverse colostomy than loop ileostomy: a prospective randomized clinical trial. Br J Surg. 2001;88(3):360–3.

Gooszen AW, Geelkerken RH, Hermans J, Lagaay MB, Gooszen HG. Temporary decompression after colorectal surgery: randomized comparison of loop ileostomy and loop colostomy. Br J Surg. 1998;85(1):76–9.

Güenaga KF, Lustosa SA, Saad SS, Saconato H, Matos D. Ileostomy or colostomy for temporary decompression of colorectal anastomosis. Cochrane Database Syst Rev. 2007;24(1):CD004647. Review.

Harris DA, Egbeare D, Jones S, Benjamin H, Woodward A, Foster ME. Complications and mortality following stoma formation. Ann R Coll Surg Engl. 2005;87(6):427–31.

Jamieson GG. The anatomy of general surgical operations. 2nd ed. Edinburgh: Churchill Livingston; 2006.

Law WL, Chu KW, Choi HK. Randomized clinical trial comparing loop ileostomy and loop transverse colostomy for faecal diversion following total mesorectal excision. Br J Surg. 2002;89(6):704–8.

Lertsithichai P, Rattanapichart P. Temporary ileostomy versus temporary colostomy: a meta-analysis of complications. Asian J Surg. 2004;27(3):202–10. Discussion 211–2.

Mileski WJ, Rege RV, Joehl RJ, Nahrwold DL. Rates of morbidity and mortality after closure of loop and end colostomy. Surg Gynecol Obstet. 1990;171(1):17–21.

Pearl RK, Prasad ML, Orsay CP, Abcarian H, Tan AB, Melzl MT. Early local complications from intestinal stomas. Arch Surg. 1985;120(10):1145–7.

Pokorny H, Herkner H, Jakesz R, Herbst F. Predictors for complications after loop stoma closure in patients with rectal cancer. World J Surg. 2006;30(8):1488–93.

Robertson I, Leung E, Hughes D, Spiers M, Donnelly L, Mackenzie I, Macdonald A. Prospective analysis of stoma-related complications. Colorectal Dis. 2005;7(3):279–85.

Sakai Y, Nelson H, Larson D, Maidl L, Young-Fadok T, Ilstrup D. Temporary transverse colostomy vs loop ileostomy in diversion: a case-matched study. Arch Surg. 2001;136(3):338–42.

Shellito PC. Complications of abdominal stoma surgery. Dis Colon Rectum. 1998;41(12):1562–72. Review.

Williams NS, Nasmyth DG, Jones D, Smith AH. De-functioning stomas: a prospective controlled trial comparing loop ileostomy with loop transverse colostomy. Br J Surg. 1986;73(7):566–70.

Right Hemicolectomy (Colostomy and Ileostomy Without Primary Anastomosis)

Ansari MZ, Collopy BT, Hart WG, Carson NJ, Chandraraj EJ. In-hospital mortality and associated complications after bowel surgery in Victorian public hospitals. ANZ J Surg. 2000;70(1):6–10.

Basili G, Lorenzetti L, Biondi G, Preziuso E, Angrisano C, Carnesecchi P, Roberto E, Goletti O. Colorectal cancer in the elderly. Is there a role for safe and curative surgery? ANZ J Surg. 2008;78(6):466–70.

Blumetti J, Luu M, Sarosi G, Hartless K, McFarlin J, Parker B, Dineen S, Huerta S, Asolati M, Varela E, Anthony T. Surgical site infections after colorectal surgery: do risk factors vary depending on the type of infection considered? Surgery. 2007;142(5):704–11.

Buchs NC, Gervaz P, Bucher P, Huber O, Mentha G, Morel P. Lessons learned from one thousand consecutive colonic resections in a teaching hospital. Swiss Med Wkly. 2007;137(17–18): 259–64.

Caricato M, Ausania F, Ripetti V, Bartolozzi F, Campoli G, Coppola R. Retrospective analysis of long-term defunctioning stoma complications after colorectal surgery. Colorectal Dis. 2007;9(6):559–61.

Harris DA, Egbeare D, Jones S, Benjamin H, Woodward A, Foster ME. Complications and mortality following stoma formation. Ann R Coll Surg Engl. 2005;87(6):427–31.

Jamieson GG. The anatomy of general surgical operations. 2nd ed. Edinburgh: Churchill Livingston; 2006.

Konishi T, Watanabe T, Kishimoto J, Nagawa H. Elective colon and rectal surgery differ in risk factors for wound infection: results of prospective surveillance. Ann Surg. 2006;244(5): 758–63.

Lipska MA, Bissett IP, Parry BR, Merrie AE. Anastomotic leakage after lower gastrointestinal anastomosis: men are at a higher risk. ANZ J Surg. 2006;76(7):579–85.

Ng SS, Lee JF, Yiu RY, Li JC, Leung WW, Leung KL. Emergency laparoscopic-assisted versus open right hemicolectomy for obstructing right-sided colonic carcinoma: a comparative study of short-term clinical outcomes. World J Surg. 2008;32(3):454–8.

Pearl RK, Prasad ML, Orsay CP, Abcarian H, Tan AB, Melzl MT. Early local complications from intestinal stomas. Arch Surg. 1985;120(10):1145–7.

Semmens JB, Platell C, Threlfall TJ, Holman CD. A population-based study of the incidence, mortality and outcomes in patients following surgery for colorectal cancer in Western Australia. ANZ J Surg. 2000;70:11–8.

Shellito PC. Complications of abdominal stoma surgery. Dis Colon Rectum. 1998;41(12):1562–72. Review.

Wyrzykowski AD, Feliciano DV, George TA, Tremblay LN, Rozycki GS, Murphy TW, Dente CJ. Emergent right hemicolectomies. Am Surg. 2005;71(8):653–6. Discussion 656–7.

Right Hemicolectomy (with Primary Ileocolonic Anastomosis)

Ansari MZ, Collopy BT, Hart WG, Carson NJ, Chandraraj EJ. In-hospital mortality and associated complications after bowel surgery in Victorian public hospitals. ANZ J Surg. 2000;70(1): 6–10.

Anwar S, Hughes S, Eadie AJ, Scott NA. Anastomotic technique and survival after right hemicolectomy for colorectal cancer. Surgeon. 2004;2(5):277–80.

Baća I, Perko Z, Bokan I, Mimica Z, Petricević A, Druzijanić N, Situm M. Technique and survival after laparoscopically assisted right hemicolectomy. Surg Endosc. 2005;19(5):650–5.

Basili G, Lorenzetti L, Biondi G, Preziuso E, Angrisano C, Carnesecchi P, Roberto E, Goletti O. Colorectal cancer in the elderly. Is there a role for safe and curative surgery? ANZ J Surg. 2008;78(6):466–70.

Blumetti J, Luu M, Sarosi G, Hartless K, McFarlin J, Parker B, Dineen S, Huerta S, Asolati M, Varela E, Anthony T. Surgical site infections after colorectal surgery: do risk factors vary depending on the type of infection considered? Surgery. 2007;142(5):704–11.

Buchs NC, Gervaz P, Bucher P, Huber O, Mentha G, Morel P. Lessons learned from one thousand consecutive colonic resections in a teaching hospital. Swiss Med Wkly. 2007;137(17–18): 259–64.

Franklin Jr ME, Gonzalez Jr JJ, Miter DB, Mansur JH, Trevino JM, Glass JL, Mancilla G, Abrego-Medina D. Laparoscopic right hemicolectomy for cancer: 11-year experience. Rev Gastroenterol Mex. 2004;69 Suppl 1:65–72.

Hohenberger W, Weber K, Matzel K, Papadopoulos T, Merkel S. Standardized surgery for colonic cancer: complete mesocolic excision and central ligation – technical notes and outcome. Colorectal Dis. 2009;11:354–64.

Ignjatovic D, Bergamaschi R. Venous bleeding from traction of transverse mesocolon. Am J Surg. 2007;194(1):141.

Jamieson GG. The anatomy of general surgical operations. 2nd ed. Edinburgh: Churchill Livingston; 2006.

Konishi T, Watanabe T, Kishimoto J, Nagawa H. Elective colon and rectal surgery differ in risk factors for wound infection: results of prospective surveillance. Ann Surg. 2006;244(5):758–63.

Lipska MA, Bissett IP, Parry BR, Merrie AE. Anastomotic leakage after lower gastrointestinal anastomosis: men are at a higher risk. ANZ J Surg. 2006;76(7):579–85.

Miller PR, Chang MC, Hoth JJ, Holmes 4th JH, Meredith JW. Colonic resection in the setting of damage control laparotomy: is delayed anastomosis safe? Am Surg. 2007;73(6):606–9. Discussion 609–10.

Minopoulos GI, Lyratzopoulos N, Efremidou HI, Romanidis K, Koujoumtzi I, Manolas KJ. Emergency operations for carcinoma of the colon. Tech Coloproctol. 2004;8 Suppl 1:s235–7.

Ng SS, Lee JF, Yiu RY, Li JC, Leung WW, Leung KL. Emergency laparoscopic-assisted versus open right hemicolectomy for obstructing right-sided colonic carcinoma: a comparative study of short-term clinical outcomes. World J Surg. 2008;32(3):454–8.

Scharfenberg M, Raue W, Junghans T, Schwenk W. "Fast-track" rehabilitation after colonic surgery in elderly patients–is it feasible? Int J Colorectal Dis. 2007;22(12):1469–74.

Semmens JB, Platell C, Threlfall TJ, Holman CD. A population-based study of the incidence, mortality and outcomes in patients following surgery for colorectal cancer in Western Australia. ANZ J Surg. 2000;70:11–8.

Tewari M, Shukla HS. Right colectomy with isoperistaltic side-to-side stapled ileocolic anastomosis. J Surg Oncol. 2005;89(2):99–101.

Tytherleigh MG, Bokey L, Chapuis PH, Dent OF. Is a minor clinical anastomotic leak clinically significant after resection of colorectal cancer? J Am Coll Surg. 2007;205(5):648–53.

Wyrzykowski AD, Feliciano DV, George TA, Tremblay LN, Rozycki GS, Murphy TW, Dente CJ. Emergent right hemicolectomies. Am Surg. 2005;71(8):653–6. Discussion 656–7.

Elective Hartmann's Procedure

Ansari MZ, Collopy BT, Hart WG, Carson NJ, Chandraraj EJ. In-hospital mortality and associated complications after bowel surgery in Victorian public hospitals. ANZ J Surg. 2000;70(1):6–10.

Basili G, Lorenzetti L, Biondi G, Preziuso E, Angrisano C, Carnesecchi P, Roberto E, Goletti O. Colorectal cancer in the elderly. Is there a role for safe and curative surgery? ANZ J Surg. 2008;78(6):466–70.

Blumetti J, Luu M, Sarosi G, Hartless K, McFarlin J, Parker B, Dineen S, Huerta S, Asolati M, Varela E, Anthony T. Surgical site infections after colorectal surgery: do risk factors vary depending on the type of infection considered? Surgery. 2007;142(5):704–11.

Buchs NC, Gervaz P, Bucher P, Huber O, Mentha G, Morel P. Lessons learned from one thousand consecutive colonic resections in a teaching hospital. Swiss Med Wkly. 2007;137(17–18):259–64.

Caricato M, Ausania F, Ripetti V, Bartolozzi F, Campoli G, Coppola R. Retrospective analysis of long-term defunctioning stoma complications after colorectal surgery. Colorectal Dis. 2007;9(6):559–61.

Harris DA, Egbeare D, Jones S, Benjamin H, Woodward A, Foster ME. Complications and mortality following stoma formation. Ann R Coll Surg Engl. 2005;87(6):427–31.

Ignjatovic D, Bergamaschi R. Venous bleeding from traction of transverse mesocolon. Am J Surg. 2007;194(1):141.

Jamieson GG. The anatomy of general surgical operations. 2nd ed. Edinburgh: Churchill Livingston; 2006.

Konishi T, Watanabe T, Kishimoto J, Nagawa H. Elective colon and rectal surgery differ in risk factors for wound infection: results of prospective surveillance. Ann Surg. 2006;244(5): 758–63.

Ret Dávalos ML, De Cicco C, D'Hoore A, De Decker B, Koninckx PR. Outcome after rectum or sigmoid resection: a review for gynecologists. J Minim Invasive Gynecol. 2007;14(1):33–8. Review.

Scharfenberg M, Raue W, Junghans T, Schwenk W. "Fast-track" rehabilitation after colonic surgery in elderly patients–is it feasible? Int J Colorectal Dis. 2007;22(12):1469–74.

Semmens JB, Platell C, Threlfall TJ, Holman CD. A population-based study of the incidence, mortality and outcomes in patients following surgery for colorectal cancer in Western Australia. ANZ J Surg. 2000;70:11–8.

Emergency Hartmann's Procedure

Ansari MZ, Collopy BT, Hart WG, Carson NJ, Chandraraj EJ. In-hospital mortality and associated complications after bowel surgery in Victorian public hospitals. ANZ J Surg. 2000;70(1): 6–10.

Basili G, Lorenzetti L, Biondi G, Preziuso E, Angrisano C, Carnesecchi P, Roberto F, Goletti O. Colorectal cancer in the elderly. Is there a role for safe and curative surgery? ANZ J Surg. 2008;78(6):466–70.

Blumetti J, Luu M, Sarosi G, Hartless K, McFarlin J, Parker B, Dineen S, Huerta S, Asolati M, Varela E, Anthony T. Surgical site infections after colorectal surgery: do risk factors vary depending on the type of infection considered? Surgery. 2007;142(5):704–11.

Buchs NC, Gervaz P, Bucher P, Huber O, Mentha G, Morel P. Lessons learned from one thousand consecutive colonic resections in a teaching hospital. Swiss Med Wkly. 2007;137(17–18): 259–64.

Caricato M, Ausania F, Ripetti V, Bartolozzi F, Campoli G, Coppola R. Retrospective analysis of long-term defunctioning stoma complications after colorectal surgery. Colorectal Dis. 2007;9(6):559–61.

Harris DA, Egbeare D, Jones S, Benjamin H, Woodward A, Foster ME. Complications and mortality following stoma formation. Ann R Coll Surg Engl. 2005;87(6):427–31.

Jamieson GG. The anatomy of general surgical operations. 2nd ed. Edinburgh: Churchill Livingston; 2006.

Ret Dávalos ML, De Cicco C, D'Hoore A, De Decker B, Koninckx PR. Outcome after rectum or sigmoid resection: a review for gynecologists. J Minim Invasive Gynecol. 2007;14(1):33–8. Review.

Scharfenberg M, Raue W, Junghans T, Schwenk W. "Fast-track" rehabilitation after colonic surgery in elderly patients–is it feasible? Int J Colorectal Dis. 2007;22(12):1469–74.

Semmens JB, Platell C, Threlfall TJ, Holman CD. A population-based study of the incidence, mortality and outcomes in patients following surgery for colorectal cancer in Western Australia. ANZ J Surg. 2000;70:11–8.

Segmental Colonic Resection (Colostomy <u>Without</u> Primary Anastomosis)

Ansari MZ, Collopy BT, Hart WG, Carson NJ, Chandraraj EJ. In-hospital mortality and associated complications after bowel surgery in Victorian public hospitals. ANZ J Surg. 2000;70(1):6–10.

Basili G, Lorenzetti L, Biondi G, Preziuso E, Angrisano C, Carnesecchi P, Roberto E, Goletti O. Colorectal cancer in the elderly. Is there a role for safe and curative surgery? ANZ J Surg. 2008;78(6):466–70.

Blumetti J, Luu M, Sarosi G, Hartless K, McFarlin J, Parker B, Dineen S, Huerta S, Asolati M, Varela E, Anthony T. Surgical site infections after colorectal surgery: do risk factors vary depending on the type of infection considered? Surgery. 2007;142(5):704–11.

Buchs NC, Gervaz P, Bucher P, Huber O, Mentha G, Morel P. Lessons learned from one thousand consecutive colonic resections in a teaching hospital. Swiss Med Wkly. 2007;137(17–18): 259–64.

Caricato M, Ausania F, Ripetti V, Bartolozzi F, Campoli G, Coppola R. Retrospective analysis of long-term defunctioning stoma complications after colorectal surgery. Colorectal Dis. 2007;9(6):559–61.

Harris DA, Egbeare D, Jones S, Benjamin H, Woodward A, Foster ME. Complications and mortality following stoma formation. Ann R Coll Surg Engl. 2005;87(6):427–31.

Jamieson GG. The anatomy of general surgical operations. 2nd ed. Edinburgh: Churchill Livingston; 2006.

Konishi T, Watanabe T, Kishimoto J, Nagawa H. Elective colon and rectal surgery differ in risk factors for wound infection: results of prospective surveillance. Ann Surg. 2006;244(5): 758–63.

Ret Dávalos ML, De Cicco C, D'Hoore A, De Decker B, Koninckx PR. Outcome after rectum or sigmoid resection: a review for gynecologists. J Minim Invasive Gynecol. 2007;14(1):33–8. Review.

Scharfenberg M, Raue W, Junghans T, Schwenk W. "Fast-track" rehabilitation after colonic surgery in elderly patients–is it feasible? Int J Colorectal Dis. 2007;22(12):1469–74.

Semmens JB, Platell C, Threlfall TJ, Holman CD. A population-based study of the incidence, mortality and outcomes in patients following surgery for colorectal cancer in Western Australia. ANZ J Surg. 2000;70:11–8.

Segmental Colonic Resection (with Primary Colonic Anastomosis)

Ansari MZ, Collopy BT, Hart WG, Carson NJ, Chandraraj EJ. In-hospital mortality and associated complications after bowel surgery in Victorian public hospitals. ANZ J Surg. 2000;70(1): 6–10.

Basili G, Lorenzetti L, Biondi G, Preziuso E, Angrisano C, Carnesecchi P, Roberto E, Goletti O. Colorectal cancer in the elderly. Is there a role for safe and curative surgery? ANZ J Surg. 2008;78(6):466–70.

Blumetti J, Luu M, Sarosi G, Hartless K, McFarlin J, Parker B, Dineen S, Huerta S, Asolati M, Varela E, Anthony T. Surgical site infections after colorectal surgery: do risk factors vary depending on the type of infection considered? Surgery. 2007;142(5):704–11.

Buchs NC, Gervaz P, Bucher P, Huber O, Mentha G, Morel P. Lessons learned from one thousand consecutive colonic resections in a teaching hospital. Swiss Med Wkly. 2007;137(17–18): 259–64.

Ignjatovic D, Bergamaschi R. Venous bleeding from traction of transverse mesocolon. Am J Surg. 2007;194(1):141.

Jamieson GG. The anatomy of general surgical operations. 2nd ed. Edinburgh: Churchill Livingston; 2006.

Köckerling F, Schneider C, Reymond MA, Scheidbach H, Scheuerlein H, Konradt J, Bruch HP, Zornig C, Köhler L, Bärlehner E, Kuthe A, Szinicz G, Richter HA, Hohenberger W. Laparoscopic resection of sigmoid diverticulitis. Results of a multicenter study. Laparoscopic Colorectal Surgery Study Group. Surg Endosc. 1999;13(6):567–71.

Konishi T, Watanabe T, Kishimoto J, Nagawa H. Elective colon and rectal surgery differ in risk factors for wound infection: results of prospective surveillance. Ann Surg. 2006;244(5): 758–63.

Peeters KC, Tollenaar RA, Marijnen CA, Klein Kranenbarg E, Steup WH, Wiggers T, Rutten HJ, van de Velde CJ, Dutch Colorectal Cancer Group. Risk factors for anastomotic failure after total mesorectal excision of rectal cancer. Br J Surg. 2005;92(2):211–6.

Pronio A, Di Filippo A, Narilli P, Mancini B, Caporilli D, Piroli S, Vestri A, Montesani C. Anastomotic dehiscence in colorectal surgery. Analysis of 1290 patients. Chir Ital. 2007;59(5):599–609. Italian.

Ret Dávalos ML, De Cicco C, D'Hoore A, De Decker B, Koninckx PR. Outcome after rectum or sigmoid resection: a review for gynecologists. J Minim Invasive Gynecol. 2007;14(1):33–8. Review.

Scharfenberg M, Raue W, Junghans T, Schwenk W. "Fast-track" rehabilitation after colonic surgery in elderly patients–is it feasible? Int J Colorectal Dis. 2007;22(12):1469–74.

Semmens JB, Platell C, Threlfall TJ, Holman CD. A population-based study of the incidence, mortality and outcomes in patients following surgery for colorectal cancer in Western Australia. ANZ J Surg. 2000;70:11–8.

Tytherleigh MG, Bokey L, Chapuis PH, Dent OF. Is a minor clinical anastomotic leak clinically significant after resection of colorectal cancer? J Am Coll Surg. 2007;205(5):648–53.

Zapletal C, Woeste G, Bechstein WO, Wullstein C. Laparoscopic sigmoid resections for diverticulitis complicated by abscesses or fistulas. Int J Colorectal Dis. 2007;22(12):1515–21.

Anterior Resection (Rectosigmoidectomy) (with or Without Loop Ileostomy)

Ansari MZ, Collopy BT, Hart WG, Carson NJ, Chandraraj EJ. In-hospital mortality and associated complications after bowel surgery in Victorian public hospitals. ANZ J Surg. 2000;70(1): 6–10.

Basili G, Lorenzetti L, Biondi G, Preziuso E, Angrisano C, Carnesecchi P, Roberto E, Goletti O. Colorectal cancer in the elderly. Is there a role for safe and curative surgery? ANZ J Surg. 2008;78(6):466–70.

Brigand C, Rohr S, Meyer C. Colorectal stapled anastomosis: results after anterior resection of the rectum for cancer. Ann Chir. 2004;129(8):427–32. French.

Enker WE, Merchant N, Cohen AM, Lanouette NM, Swallow C, Guillem J, Paty P, Minsky B, Weyrauch K, Quan SH. Safety and efficacy of low anterior resection for rectal cancer: 681 consecutive cases from a specialty service. Ann Surg. 1999;230(4):544–52. Discussion 552–4.

Jamieson GG. The anatomy of general surgical operations. 2nd ed. Edinburgh: Churchill Livingston; 2006.

Kanellos I, Vasiliadis K, Angelopoulos S, Tsachalis T, Pramateftakis MG, Mantzoros I, Betsis D. Anastomotic leakage following anterior resection for rectal cancer. Tech Coloproctol. 2004;8 Suppl 1:s79–81.

Law WI, Chu KW, Ho JW, Chan CW. Risk factors for anastomotic leakage after low anterior resection with total mesorectal excision. Am J Surg. 2000;179(2):92–6.

Lyall A, Mc Adam TK, Townend J, Loudon MA. Factors affecting anastomotic complications following anterior resection in rectal cancer. Colorectal Dis. 2007;9(9):801–7.

Matthiessen P, Hallböök O, Andersson M, Rutegård J, Sjödahl R. Risk factors for anastomotic leakage after anterior resection of the rectum. Colorectal Dis. 2004;6(6):462–9.

Rodríguez-Ramírez SE, Uribe A, Ruiz-García EB, Labastida S, Luna-Pérez P. Risk factors for anastomotic leakage after preoperative chemoradiation therapy and low anterior resection with total mesorectal excision for locally advanced rectal cancer. Rev Invest Clin. 2006; 58(3):204–10.

Semmens JB, Platell C, Threlfall TJ, Holman CD. A population-based study of the incidence, mortality and outcomes in patients following surgery for colorectal cancer in Western Australia. ANZ J Surg. 2000;70:11–8.

Vermeulen J, Lange JF, van der Harst E. Impaired anastomotic healing after preoperative radiotherapy followed by anterior resection for treatment of rectal carcinoma. S Afr J Surg. 2006;44(1):12–14–6.

Restoration of Continuity

Aydin HN, Remzi FH, Tekkis PP, Fazio VW. Hartmann's reversal is associated with high postoperative adverse events. Dis Colon Rectum. 2005;48(11):2117–26.

Bakx R, Busch OR, Bemelman WA, Veldink GJ, Slors JF, van Lanschot JJ. Morbidity of temporary loop ileostomies. Dig Surg. 2004;21(4):277–81.

Bell C, Asolati M, Hamilton E, Fleming J, Nwariaku F, Sarosi G, Anthony T. A comparison of complications associated with colostomy reversal versus ileostomy reversal. Am J Surg. 2005;190(5):717–20.

Caricato M, Ausania F, Ripetti V, Bartolozzi F, Campoli G, Coppola R. Retrospective analysis of long-term defunctioning stoma complications after colorectal surgery. Colorectal Dis. 2007;9(6):559–61.

Güenaga KF, Lustosa SA, Saad SS, Saconato H, Matos D. Ileostomy or colostomy for temporary decompression of colorectal anastomosis. Cochrane Database Syst Rev. 2007;24(1):CD004647. Review.

Harris DA, Egbeare D, Jones S, Benjamin H, Woodward A, Foster ME. Complications and mortality following stoma formation. Ann R Coll Surg Engl. 2005;87(6):427–31.

Jamieson GG. The anatomy of general surgical operations. 2nd ed. Edinburgh: Churchill Livingston; 2006.

Kaidar-Person O, Person B, Wexner SD. Complications of construction and closure of temporary loop ileostomy. J Am Coll Surg. 2005;201(5):759–73.

Keck JO, Collopy BT, Ryan PJ, Fink R, Mackay JR, Woods RJ. Reversal of Hartmann's procedure: effect of timing and technique on ease and safety. Dis Colon Rectum. 1994;37(3):243–8. Review.

Lahat G, Tulchinsky H, Goldman G, Klauzner JM, Rabau M. Wound infection after ileostomy closure: a prospective randomized study comparing primary vs. delayed primary closure techniques. Tech Coloproctol. 2005;9(3):206–8.

Lertsithichai P, Rattanapichart P. Temporary ileostomy versus temporary colostomy: a meta-analysis of complications. Asian J Surg. 2004;27(3):202–10. Discussion 211–2.

Perez RO, Habr-Gama A, Seid VE, Proscurshim I, Sousa Jr AH, Kiss DR, Linhares M, Sapucahy M, Gama-Rodrigues J. Loop ileostomy morbidity: timing of closure matters. Dis Colon Rectum. 2006;49(10):1539–45.

Pokorny H, Herkner H, Jakesz R, Herbst F. Predictors for complications after loop stoma closure in patients with rectal cancer. World J Surg. 2006;30(8):1488–93.

Rathnayake MM, Kumarage SK, Wijesuriya SR, Munasinghe BN, Ariyaratne MH, Deen KI. Complications of loop ileostomy and ileostomy closure and their implications for extended enterostomal therapy: a prospective clinical audit. Int J Nurs Stud. 2008;45(8):1118–21.

Robertson I, Leung E, Hughes D, Spiers M, Donnelly L, Mackenzie I, Macdonald A. Prospective analysis of stoma-related complications. Colorectal Dis. 2005;7(3):279–85.

Rosen MJ, Cobb WS, Kercher KW, Heniford BT. Laparoscopic versus open colostomy reversal: a comparative analysis. J Gastrointest Surg. 2006;10(6):895–900.

Shellito PC. Complications of abdominal stoma surgery. Dis Colon Rectum. 1998;41(12):1562–72. Review.

Williams LA, Sagar PM, Finan PJ, Burke D. The outcome of loop ileostomy closure: a prospective study. Colorectal Dis. 2008;10(5):460–4.

Abdominoperineal Resection of the Rectum

Ansari MZ, Collopy BT, Hart WG, Carson NJ, Chandraraj EJ. In-hospital mortality and associated complications after bowel surgery in Victorian public hospitals. ANZ J Surg. 2000;70(1): 6–10.

Araujo SE, Jr Da Silva eSousa AH, de Campos FG, Habr-Gama A, Dumarco RB, Caravatto PP, Nahas SC, da Silva J, Kiss DR, Gama-Rodrigues JJ. Conventional approach to laparoscopic abdominoperineal resection for rectal cancer treatment after neoadjuvant chemoradiation: results of a prospective randomized trial. Rev Hosp Clin Fac Med Sao Paulo. 2003;58(3): 133–40.

Aziz O, Constantinides V, Tekkis PP, Athanasiou T, Purkayastha S, Paraskeva P, Darzi AW, Heriot AG. Laparoscopic versus open surgery for rectal cancer: a meta-analysis. Ann Surg Oncol. 2006;13(3):413–24.

Basili G, Lorenzetti L, Biondi G, Preziuso E, Angrisano C, Carnesecchi P, Roberto E, Goletti O. Colorectal cancer in the elderly. Is there a role for safe and curative surgery? ANZ J Surg. 2008;78(6):466–70.

Christian CK, Kwaan MR, Betensky RA, Breen EM, Zinner MJ, Bleday R. Risk factors for perineal wound complications following abdominoperineal resection. Dis Colon Rectum. 2005; 48(1):43–8.

Gao F, Cao YF, Chen LS. Meta-analysis of short-term outcomes after laparoscopic resection for rectal cancer. Int J Colorectal Dis. 2006;21(7):652–6.

Jamieson GG. The anatomy of general surgical operations. 2nd ed. Edinburgh: Churchill Livingston; 2006.

Luna-Pérez P, Rodríguez-Ramírez S, Vega J, Sandoval E, Labastida S. Morbidity and mortality following abdominoperineal resection for low rectal adenocarcinoma. Rev Invest Clin. 2001;53(5):388–95. Review.

Semmens JB, Platell C, Threlfall TJ, Holman CD. A population-based study of the incidence, mortality and outcomes in patients following surgeryfor colorectal cancer in Western Australia. ANZ J Surg. 2000;70:11–8.

Wong DC, Chung CC, Chan ES, Kwok AS, Tsang WW, Li MK. Laparoscopic abdominoperineal resection revisited: are there any health-related benefits? A comparative study. Tech Coloproctol. 2006;10(1):37–42.

Wu WX, Sun YM, Hua YB, Shen LZ. Laparoscopic versus conventional open resection of rectal carcinoma: a clinical comparative study. World J Gastroenterol. 2004;10(8):1167–70.

Total Procto-Colectomy and Restorative Ileo-Anal (or Ilio-Rectal) Pouch Reconstruction

Ansari MZ, Collopy BT, Hart WG, Carson NJ, Chandraraj EJ. In-hospital mortality and associated complications after bowel surgery in Victorian public hospitals. ANZ J Surg. 2000;70(1): 6–10.

Basili G, Lorenzetti L, Biondi G, Preziuso E, Angrisano C, Carnesecchi P, Roberto E, Goletti O. Colorectal cancer in the elderly. Is there a role for safe and curative surgery? ANZ J Surg. 2008;78(6):466–70.

Brigand C, Rohr S, Meyer C. Colorectal stapled anastomosis: results after anterior resection of the rectum for cancer. Ann Chir. 2004;129(8):427–32. French.

Cozzi P. Improving cancer control and recovery of potency after radical prostatectomy: nerve sparing versus nerve resection with grafting. ANZ J Surg. 2008;78:834–5.

Enker WE, Merchant N, Cohen AM, Lanouette NM, Swallow C, Guillem J, Paty P, Minsky B, Weyrauch K, Quan SH. Safety and efficacy of low anterior resection for rectal cancer: 681 consecutive cases from a specialty service. Ann Surg. 1999;230(4):544–52. Discussion 552–4.

Jamieson GG. The anatomy of general surgical operations. 2nd ed. Edinburgh: Churchill Livingston; 2006.

Kanellos I, Vasiliadis K, Angelopoulos S, Tsachalis T, Pramateftakis MG, Mantzoros I, Betsis D. Anastomotic leakage following anterior resection for rectal cancer. Tech Coloproctol. 2004;8 Suppl 1:s79–81.

Law WI, Chu KW, Ho JW, Chan CW. Risk factors for anastomotic leakage after low anterior resection with total mesorectal excision. Am J Surg. 2000;179(2):92–6.

Lyall A, Mc Adam TK, Townend J, Loudon MA. Factors affecting anastomotic complications following anterior resection in rectal cancer. Colorectal Dis. 2007;9(9):801–7.

Matthiessen P, Hallböök O, Andersson M, Rutegård J, Sjödahl R. Risk factors for anastomotic leakage after anterior resection of the rectum. Colorectal Dis. 2004;6(6):462–9.

Rodríguez-Ramírez SE, Uribe A, Ruiz-García EB, Labastida S, Luna-Pérez P. Risk factors for anastomotic leakage after preoperative chemoradiation therapy and low anterior resection with total mesorectal excision for locally advanced rectal cancer. Rev Invest Clin. 2006;58(3):204–10.

Semmens JB, Platell C, Threlfall TJ, Holman CD. A population-based study of the incidence, mortality and outcomes in patients following surgeryfor colorectal cancer in Western Australia. ANZ J Surg. 2000;70:11–8.

Vermeulen J, Lange JF, van der Harst E. Impaired anastomotic healing after preoperative radiotherapy followed by anterior resection for treatment of rectal carcinoma. S Afr J Surg. 2006;44(1):12. 14–6.

Chapter 3
Anal Surgery

Bruce Waxman and Brendon J. Coventry

General Perspective and Overview

Anorectal problems are among the most common problems that occur on a regular basis in general surgery and also can prove to be among the most challenging. The spectrum is broad ranging from minor anal leakage and pruritus to deep ischiorectal abscesses with associated multiple transsphincteric fistulae.

Fecal incontinence is not uncommon immediately after surgery, especially in the elderly, but is often a major problem if it is persistent past several days postoperatively. Avoidance of excessive dilatation of the anal sphincters is essential to reduce the risk of incontinence.

Recurrent anal problems can also be a significant challenge for the surgeon and very difficult for the patient. Use of aperients can be particularly helpful for the patient (and surgeon) postoperatively after anal surgery. Advising the patient to avoid constipation is often very helpful to reduce the risk of further hemorrhoids or fissures from occurring. Careful use of constipating agents, especially narcotics, is often helpful in avoiding constipation postoperatively, from almost any surgery where pain control is an issue. Recurrent, difficult, or high fistulae are usually best dealt with by assessment from a specialist colorectal surgeon and preferably early in the course of management.

With these factors and facts in mind, the information given in these chapters must be interpreted appropriately and discernibly.

B. Waxman, BMedSc, MBBS, FRACS, FRCS(Eng), FACS (✉)
Academic Surgical Unit, Monash University, Monash Health
and Southern Clinical School, Dandenong, VIC, Australia
e-mail: bruce.waxman@southernhealth.org.au

B.J. Coventry, BMBS, PhD, FRACS, FACS, FRSM
Discipline of Surgery, Royal Adelaide Hospital, University of Adelaide,
L5 Eleanor Harrald Building, North Terrace, 5000 Adelaide, SA, Australia

B.J. Coventry (ed.), *Lower Abdominal and Perineal Surgery*,
Surgery: Complications, Risks and Consequences,
DOI 10.1007/978-1-4471-5469-3_3, © Springer-Verlag London 2014

The **use of specialized colorectal units with standardized preoperative assessment, multidisciplinary input, and high-quality postoperative care** is essential to the success of complex anal surgery overall and can significantly reduce risk of complications or aid early detection, prompt intervention, and cost.

Important Note

It should be emphasized that the risks and frequencies that are given here *represent derived figures*. These *figures are best estimates of relative frequencies across most institutions*, not merely the highest-performing ones, and as such are often representative of a number of studies, which include different patients with differing comorbidities and different surgeons. In addition, the risks of complications in lower- or higher-risk patients may lie outside these estimated ranges, and individual clinical judgment is required as to the expected risks communicated to the patient and staff or for other purposes. The range of risks is also derived from experience and the literature; while risks outside this range may exist, certain risks may be reduced or absent due to variations of procedures or surgical approaches. It is recognized that different patients, practitioners, institutions, regions, and countries may vary in their requirements and recommendations.

Examination Under Anesthesia (EUA) (+/− Anal Dilatation)

Description

General anesthetic is usually used complemented with local anesthetic infiltration. The lithotomy position is used to examine the perianal region, anus, and lower rectum. Some surgeons prefer the prone jackknife position. The procedure involves careful inspection, including parting the buttocks, digital examination with the index finger, and sigmoidoscopic and/or proctoscopic (anoscopic) examination of the lower rectum. Use of a headlight improves illumination particularly when using the anoscope.

The presence of hemorrhoids, excessive or loose anal tone, induration, masses, tenderness, fissures, fistulae, blood, mucus, pus, or rectal tumors is noted. Anteriorly, examination of the prostate in the male, and cervix in the female, is also essential. In some cases, a combined rectal and vaginal examination may be useful in defining a rectovaginal fistula.

Mild anal dilatation may occur if a speculum/anoscope is used, such as the Fansler, Eisenhammer, or Parkes anoscopes, but intentional manual anal dilatation carries the risk of incontinence due to over-stretching of the anal sphincter, especially in the elderly.

Table 3.1 Examination under anesthesia (+/− anal dilatation) estimated frequency of complications, risks, and consequences

Complications, risks, and consequences	Estimated frequency
Most significant/serious complications	
Fecal incontinence	
Transient	50–80 %
Longer term/soiling (rare)[a, b]	1–5 %
Bleeding (acute fissure formation)[a]	5–20 %
Rare significant/serious problems	
Missed pathology[a]	0.1–1 %
Infection	0.1–1 %
Less serious complications	
Pain on passage of bowel actions (initially)[a]	50–80 %
Urinary retention/catheterization (males)	0.1–1 %

[a]Dependent on underlying pathology, anatomy, surgical technique, and preferences
[b]The degree of anal dilatation is associated with higher risk of incontinence

Anatomical Points

The anus has two circular muscles, the internal sphincter (involuntary muscle) and the external sphincter (voluntary muscle) which control muscle tone and fecal/gas control, respectively. The anal cushions are transposed in the 3, 7, and 11 o'clock positions (12 o'clock being anterior) around the anus and carry blood vessels, which can become enlarged and engorged as hemorrhoidal tissue.

Perspective

See Table 3.1. The complications from a simple EUA are minimal and the benefits are maximal in obtaining a good pain-free inspection and a more accurate diagnosis.

Major Complications

The main potential problem is **incontinence**, but usually only if an intentional anal dilatation is performed. Other complications are usually minor. Occasionally, **anal pain** may be significant if an anal fissure is diagnosed at the EUA.

Consent and Risk Reduction

Main Points to Explain

- Discomfort
- Bleeding
- Fecal incontinence
- Risks without surgery

Perianal Abscess Drainage

Description

General anesthesia is usually used, but on occasions local anesthesia may be used. GA affords better examination of the anus and palpation of the sphincter muscles, particularly the internal sphincter.

The lithotomy or prone jackknife position is used, depending on the surgeon's preference. The prone jackknife position offers a better view of the anus for the operating surgeon and reduces the edema associated with the supine position, and any bleeding usually runs away from the operating surgeon into the rectum. Anesthetists sometimes object to the prone jackknife position, because of the physiological effects on the circulatory system and respiratory system.

Views of the anal canal are greatly enhanced by the use of the operating anoscope such as the Fansler, Eisenhammer, or Parks anoscopes and the addition of a headlight.

The objective of this operation is to establish the anatomy, drain the perianal abscess, and settle the infection. In particular, the surgeon should attempt to identify the presence of an internal opening of a potential fistula at the dentate line, by general pressure on the abscess before incising the abscess.

The abscess is then drained externally, either with a simple radial incision or cruciate incision, any loculations are broken down by the finger, the cavity is lavaged with saline and/or antiseptic, and light packing of the cavity is performed with an alginate dressing. Injecting a weak solution of hydrogen peroxide may further identify an internal opening and hence a fistula.

Some colorectal surgeons prefer the use of a "mushroom" catheter placed in the abscess cavity. If an internal opening is identified, then placement of a loose seton, such as a vascular loop, may be useful. For superficial and submucosal fistulae, abscess drainage can be combined with fistulotomy (laying open).

The most common perianal abscess is either mucosal or intersphincteric indicating their communication between the skin and dentate line, the former being at the level of the submucosa and the latter being through the intersphincteric plane between the internal sphincter and the external sphincter. An ischiorectal abscess forms as an extrasphincteric abscess that has been a communication between the crypt gland level of the dentate line through both the internal and external sphincters with abscess formation in the ischiorectal fossa (see below). The more sphincter that is involved in the abscess formation, the greater the likelihood of longer-term incontinence and the need for care in performing fistulotomy at the initial operation.

Anatomical Points

The anus has two circular muscles, the internal sphincter (involuntary muscle) and the external sphincter (voluntary muscle) which control muscle tone and fecal/gas

Table 3.2 Perianal abscess drainage estimated frequency of complications, risks, and consequences

Complications, risks, and consequences	Estimated frequency
Most significant/serious complications	
Infection[a] overall	5–20 %
Subcutaneous	1–5 %
Recurrent perianal abscess	5–20 %
Systemic sepsis[a]	1–5 %
Hepatic portal sepsis (rare)	0.1–1 %
Bleeding/hematoma formation[a]	1–5 %
Pain on passage of bowel actions[a]	50–80 %
Fecal incontinence	
Transient	1–5 %
Longer term (rare)	0.1–1 %
Rare significant/serious problems	
Missed pathology[a]	0.1–1 %
Chronic ulceration with hypergranulation[a]	0.1–1 %
Multi-system organ failure (renal, pulmonary, cardiac failure)[a]	<0.1 %
Less serious complications	
Residual pain/discomfort	
Short term (<4 weeks)	50–80 %
Longer term >12 weeks	0.1–1 %
Scarring	0.1–1 %
Urinary retention/catheterization (males)	1–5 %

[a]Dependent on underlying pathology, anatomy, surgical technique, and preferences

control, respectively. The anal cushions are transposed in the 3, 7, and 11 o'clock positions (12 o'clock being anterior) around the anus and carry blood vessels, which can become enlarged and engorged as hemorrhoidal tissue. The anal (crypt) glands lie at the dentate line in the anal canal and communicate with the intersphincteric plane between the internal and external sphincters. Infection of these glands and extension into the ischiorectal fossa may occur. Abscess formation in either of these locations may be evident at the perianal skin surface.

Perspective

See Table 3.2. Subsequent fistula formation is the most common consequence of this procedure and is the cause of recurrent perianal abscess. Occasionally Fournier's gangrene may develop in association with perianal abscess, but this is most commonly associated with patients with other significant comorbidities particularly diabetes, immunosuppression, and poor general health. Fournier's gangrene is often the first presenting problem rather than as a direct postoperative complication of the perianal abscess drainage.

Major Complications

The main potential problem is **fecal incontinence**, but usually only if the external sphincter is interrupted, for example, when surgery for a high fistula is performed. Other complications are minor. Occasionally, **buttock or perianal pain** may be significant on defecation after surgery, but usually settles within 5–7 days. **Localized cellulitis, recurrent abscess formation, systemic infection,** and rarely **multisystem organ failure** can occur.

Consent and Risk Reduction

Main Points to Explain

- Discomfort
- Bleeding
- Problems with GA
- Recurrent abscess formation
- Fecal incontinence
- Infection
- Further surgery
- Risks without surgery

Ischiorectal Abscess Drainage

Description

General anesthesia is usually used, but on occasions local anesthesia may be used. GA affords better examination of the anus and palpation of the sphincter muscles, particularly the internal sphincter.

The lithotomy or prone jackknife position is used, depending on the surgeon's preference. The prone jackknife position offers a better view of the anus for the operating surgeon and reduces the edema associated with the supine position, and any bleeding usually runs away from the operating surgeon into the rectum. Anesthetists sometimes object to the prone jackknife position, because of the physiological effects on the circulatory system and respiratory system. Views of the anal canal are greatly enhanced by the use of the operating anoscope such as the Fansler, Eisenhammer, or Parks anoscopes and a headlight.

The objective of this operation is to establish the anatomy, drain the ischiorectal abscess, and settle the infection. In particular the surgeon should attempt to identify the presence of an internal opening by general pressure on the abscess before incising the abscess using an operating anoscope to view the level of the dentate line, being the likely source of the internal opening.

The abscess is then drained externally, either with a simple radial incision or cruciate incision, any loculations are broken down by the finger, the cavity is lavaged with saline antiseptic, and light packing of the cavity is performed. Injecting a weak solution of hydrogen peroxide may further identify an internal opening and hence a fistula.

Some colorectal surgeons prefer the use of a "mushroom" catheter placed in the abscess cavity. If an internal opening is identified, then placement of a loose seton, such as a vascular loop, is preferable to fistulotomy (laying open), as incision may divide the external sphincter muscle and lead to incontinence of feces.

An ischiorectal abscess forms as an extrasphincteric abscess that has been a communication between the crypt gland level of the dentate line through both the internal and external sphincter with abscess formation within the ischiorectal fossa. The more sphincter that is involved in the abscess formation, the greater the likelihood of longer-term incontinence.

Anatomical Points

The anus has two circular muscles, the internal sphincter (involuntary muscle) and the external sphincter (voluntary muscle) which control muscle tone and fecal/gas control, respectively. The anal cushions are transposed in the 3, 7, and 11 o'clock positions (12 o'clock being anterior) around the anus and carry blood vessels, which can become enlarged and engorged as hemorrhoidal sacs. The anal glands lie at the dentate line in the anal canal and communicate with the intersphincteric plane between the internal and external sphincters. Infection of these glands and extension into the ischiorectal fossa may occur. Abscess formation in either of these locations may be evident at the perianal skin surface.

Perspective

See Table 3.3. The complications for ischiorectal abscess are similar, but at a higher incidence than for perianal abscess treatment. Subsequent fistula formation is the most common consequence of this procedure and is the cause of recurrent ischiorectal abscess. Occasionally Fournier's (synergistic) gangrene may develop in association with perianal abscess, but this is most commonly associated with patients with other significant comorbidities particularly diabetes, immunosuppression, and poor general health. Fournier's gangrene is often the first presenting problem rather than as a direct postoperative complication of the perianal abscess drainage.

Major Complications

The main potential problem is **fecal incontinence**, but usually only if the external sphincter is interrupted, for example, when surgery for a high fistula is performed.

Table 3.3 Ischiorectal abscess drainage estimated frequency of complications, risks, and consequences

Complications, risks, and consequences	Estimated frequency
Most significant/serious complications	
Infection[a] overall	5–20 %
Subcutaneous	1–5 %
Intraabdominal/pelvic (peritonitis, abscess)	5–20 %
Systemic sepsis[a]	1–5 %
Hepatic portal sepsis (rare)	0.1–1 %
Bleeding/hematoma formation[a]	1–5 %
Multi-system failure (renal, pulmonary, cardiac failure)[a]	1–5 %
Pain on passage of bowel actions[a]	50–80 %
Fecal incontinence	
Transient	20–50 %
Longer term/soiling (rare)[a]	0.1–1 %
Rare significant/serious problems	
Missed pathology[a]	0.1–1 %
Chronic ulceration with hypergranulation[a]	0.1–1 %
Inadvertent high fecal/purulent fistula	0.1–1 %
Less serious complications	
Urinary retention/catheterization (males)	1–5 %
Persistent discharge	0.1–1 %
Residual pain/discomfort	
Short term (<4 weeks)	50–80 %
Longer term (>12 weeks)	0.1–1 %
Scarring	0.1–1 %

[a]Dependent on underlying pathology, anatomy, surgical technique, and preferences

Other complications are minor. Occasionally, **buttock or perianal pain** may be significant, especially on defecation after surgery, but usually settles within 5–7 days. Initial discomfort is usual after a seton has been inserted, but this usually settles quickly. **Localized cellulitis**, **recurrent abscess formation**, **systemic infection**, and rarely **severe sepsis** with **multi-system organ failure** can occur.

Consent and Risk Reduction

Main Points to Explain

- Discomfort
- Bleeding
- Problems with GA
- Failure to drain the abscess
- Recurrent abscess formation
- Infection and severe sepsis
- Fecal incontinence
- Further surgery
- Risks without surgery

Lateral Internal Sphincterotomy

Description

General anesthesia is usually used, but on occasions local anesthesia may be used. GA affords better examination of the anus and palpation of the sphincter muscles, particularly the internal sphincter.

The lithotomy or prone jackknife position is used, depending on the surgeon's preference. The prone jackknife position offers a better view of the anus for the operating surgeon and reduces the edema associated with the supine position, and any bleeding usually runs away from the operating surgeon into the rectum. Anesthetists sometimes object to the prone jackknife position, because of the physiological effects on the circulatory system and respiratory system.

Views of the anal canal are greatly enhanced by the use of the operating anoscope such as the Fansler, Eisenhammer, or Parks anoscopes and a headlight. The objective of this procedure is to carefully examine the anal canal and lower rectum to confirm the diagnosis and divide the internal sphincter by either the closed, open, or combination technique. The left lateral position is usually selected for convenience. Local (long-acting, adrenalin-containing) anesthetic infiltration may be used to define planes, reduce bleeding, and aid postoperative pain relief.

The closed technique uses a no. 11 scalpel and blade placed between the external and internal sphincters through a small skin stab incision, incising the sphincter from outside inward and completing the sphincterotomy by gentle pressure with the finger in a circumferential manner.

The open method incises the perianal skin longitudinally to expose the internal sphincter which is then divided longitudinally under direct vision, using either a scalpel, scissors, or diathermy to expose the external sphincter. The mucosa is then either sutured or left open.

The combination method makes a small radial incision, adjacent to the anal verge, to expose the external and internal sphincters and the planes either side of the internal sphincter are dissected easily with artery forceps or blunt scissors. The internal sphincter is divided using scissors and palpated with the finger to ensure adequate division. Some surgeons prefer to incise the internal sphincter in the base of a fissure; however, scarring and inflammation may make the tissue planes more difficult to define.

Anatomical Points

The anus has two circular muscles, the internal sphincter (involuntary muscle) and the external sphincter (voluntary muscle) which control muscle tone and fecal/gas control, respectively. The anal cushions are transposed in the 3, 7, and 11 o'clock positions (12 o'clock being anterior) around the anus and carry blood vessels, which

Table 3.4 Lateral internal sphincterotomy estimated frequency of complications, risks, and consequences

Complications, risks, and consequences	Estimated frequency
Most significant/serious complications	
Infection[a] overall	0.1–1 %
Subcutaneous	0.1–1 %
Perianal abscess	0.1–1 %
Systemic sepsis[a]	0.1–1 %
Hepatic portal sepsis (rare)	0.1–1 %
Bleeding/hematoma formation[a]	1–5 %
Pain on passage of bowel actions[a]	50–80 %
Fecal incontinence	
Transient	1–5 %
Longer term/soiling (rare)	0.1–1 %
Recurrence of fissure(s)[a]	5–20 %
Rare significant/serious problems	
Missed pathology[a]	0.1–1 %
Chronic ulceration with hypergranulation[a]	0.1–1 %
Anal stenosis (rare)	0.1–1 %
Multi-system failure (renal, pulmonary, cardiac failure)[a]	<0.1 %
Less serious complications	
Residual pain/discomfort	
Short term (<4 weeks)	50–80 %
Longer term (>12 weeks)	0.1–1 %
Scarring	0.1–1 %
Urinary retention/catheterization (males)	0.1–1 %

[a]Dependent on underlying pathology, anatomy, surgical technique, and preferences

can become enlarged and engorged as hemorrhoidal tissue, which may render sphincterotomy difficult. Chronic scarring or perianal sepsis may also alter the anatomy.

Perspective

See Table 3.4. Sphincterotomy for anal fissure may be performed in a tailored manner, which involves a measured sphincterotomy with division of the internal sphincter relevant to the length of the fissure rather than always dividing the internal sphincter to the dentate line. Sphincterotomy beyond the dentate line will increase the incidence of incontinence, particularly incontinence for flatus.

Bleeding is the most common immediate problem, and this usually resolves spontaneously, though perianal bruising may be a problem and extensive bleeding in the ischiorectal fossa may occasionally occur. Local cellulitis and perianal abscess may occur primarily or secondary to a hematoma. Fistula is rare. Incontinence, particularly incontinence for flatus is the most distressing initial symptom, but usually resolves. Incontinence for feces is not as common, but can occur usually resolving within weeks, but very rarely being permanent. **The potential for incontinence and its significant consequences, particularly in women, has been the driver for making this operation a lesser resort after chemical means of relaxing the internal sphincter, such as the use of nitrous oxide inhibitors, calcium channel blockers, and botulinum toxin.**

Major Complications

The main potential problem is **fecal incontinence**, but usually only if the external sphincter is interrupted, for example, when surgery deeply or above the dentate line is performed. Other complications are usually minor. Occasionally, **buttock or perianal pain** may be significant, especially on defecation after surgery, but usually settles within 5–7 days. Initial **bleeding** is usual after a sphincterotomy, but this usually settles quickly. Severe bleeding may occur but is rare, although it may require **further surgery. Localized cellulitis, abscess formation, systemic infection,** and very **rarely multi-system organ failure** can occur.

Consent and Risk Reduction

Main Points to Explain

- Discomfort
- Bleeding
- Problems with GA
- Infection
- Fecal incontinence
- Recurrent fissure
- Further surgery
- Risks without surgery

Anal Fissurectomy

Description

General anesthesia is usually used, but on occasions local anesthesia may be used. GA affords better examination of the anus and palpation of the sphincter muscles, particularly the internal sphincter.

The lithotomy or prone jackknife position is used, depending on the surgeon's preference. The prone jackknife position offers a better view of the anus for the operating surgeon and reduces the edema associated with the supine position, and any bleeding usually runs away from the operating surgeon into the rectum. Anesthetists sometimes object to the prone jackknife position, because of the physiological effects on the circulatory system and respiratory system.

Views of the anal canal are greatly enhanced by the use of the operating anoscope such as the Fansler, Eisenhammer, or Parks anoscopes and a headlight. The most common position for an anal fissure is posteriorly; however, anterior fissures are also common in females, and both can occur concurrently. The objective of this procedure is to carefully examine the anal canal and lower rectum to confirm the diagnosis and excise the anal fissure using an elliptical incision down to and exposing the internal sphincter.

Local (long-acting, adrenalin-containing) anesthetic infiltration may be used to define planes, reduce bleeding, and aid postoperative pain relief. Some surgeons prefer to incise the internal sphincter in the base of a fissure; however, scarring and inflammation may make the tissue planes difficult to define.

Anatomical Points

The anus has two circular muscles, the internal sphincter (involuntary muscle) and the external sphincter (voluntary muscle) which control muscle tone and fecal/gas control, respectively. The anal cushions are transposed in the 3, 7, and 11 o'clock positions (12 o'clock being anterior) around the anus and carry blood vessels, which can become enlarged and engorged as hemorrhoidal sacs, which may render sphincterotomy difficult. Chronic scarring or perianal sepsis may also alter the anatomy.

Perspective

See Table 3.5. Fissurectomy for anal fissure may be performed to remove the fissure; however, it does not address the problem of increased internal sphincter tone, as the underlying cause. Fissure persistence or recurrence is therefore higher than with sphincterotomy. Some surgeons prefer to also perform a sphincterotomy in the base of the fissurectomy site. Bleeding is the most common immediate problem and this usually resolves spontaneously, although perianal bruising may be a problem and extensive submucosal bleeding may occasionally occur, but it is usually visible on clothing or toilet paper. Local cellulitis and perianal abscess may occur primarily or secondary to a hematoma. Fistula is extremely rare. Continued fissure and pain is the most common problem. Incontinence, particularly incontinence for flatus can be a distressing initial symptom, but usually resolves. Incontinence for feces is very uncommon but can occur usually resolving within weeks, but very rarely being permanent due to chronic fissure and scarring.

Table 3.5 Anal fissurectomy estimated frequency of complications, risks, and consequences

Complications, risks, and consequences	Estimated frequency
Most significant/serious complications	
Infection[a] overall	0.1–1 %
Subcutaneous	0.1–1 %
Perianal abscess	0.1–1 %
Bleeding/hematoma formation[a]	1–5 %
Pain on passage of bowel actions[a]	50–80 %
Fecal incontinence	
Transient	1–5 %
Longer term (rare)	<0.1 %
Recurrence of fissure(s)[a]	5–20 %
Rare significant/serious problems	
Missed pathology[a]	0.1–1 %
Chronic ulceration with hypergranulation[a]	0.1–1 %
Anal stenosis (rare)	0.1–1 %
Less serious complications	
Residual pain/discomfort	
Short term (<4 weeks)	50–80 %
Longer term (>12 weeks)	0.1–1 %
Urinary retention/catheterization (males)	1–5 %
Scarring	0.1–1 %

[a]Dependent on underlying pathology, anatomy, surgical technique, and preferences

Major Complications

The main potential problem is **perianal pain** which may be significant, especially on defecation after surgery, but usually settles within 5–7 days. **Incontinence** to flatus can occur, as can fecal incontinence, but this is very rare. Other complications are usually minor. Initial **bleeding** is usual after fissurectomy, but this usually settles quickly. Severe bleeding may occur but is very rare, although it may require **further surgery**. **Recurrent/persistent fissure**, **localized cellulitis**, and rarely **systemic infection** can occur.

Consent and Risk Reduction

Main Points to Explain

- Discomfort
- Bleeding
- Problems with GA
- Recurrent fissure
- Fecal incontinence
- Infection
- Further surgery
- Risks without surgery

Laying Open of Anal Fistula with/Without Excision (Fistulotomy) and the LIFT (Ligation of the Intersphincteric Tract) Procedure

Description

General anesthesia is usually used, but on occasions local anesthesia may be used. GA affords better examination of the anus and palpation of the sphincter muscles, particularly the internal sphincter.

The lithotomy or prone jackknife position is used, depending on the surgeon's preference. The prone jackknife position offers a better view of the anus for the operating surgeon and reduces the edema associated with the supine position, and any bleeding usually runs away from the operating surgeon into the rectum. Anesthetists sometimes object to the prone jackknife position, because of the physiological effects on the circulatory system and respiratory system.

Views of the anal canal are greatly enhanced by the use of the operating anoscope such as the Fansler, Eisenhammer, or Parks anoscopes and a headlight.

There are five main types of fistulae: *submucosal* (superficial), *intersphincteric*, *transsphincteric*, *suprasphincteric*, and *extrasphincteric* (supralevator). Setons are often used for fistulae through or above the external sphincter, because of the high risk of causing incontinence with fistulotomy.

The objective of the *fistulotomy* operation is to convert the fistula from a tunnel into an open "gutter" allowing healing by secondary intention of the subcutaneous fatty tissue, mucosa, and skin while dividing as little sphincter muscle as possible. Superficial and intersphincteric fistulae can often be layed open easily without problems. For deep or high fistulae, a previously inserted loose seton may have been in position for 6–8 weeks, having gradually become more superficial. The fistula tract is identified with a probe or artery forceps and the tunnel laid open with diathermy. Either the tract is then curetted and may be left to heal by secondary intention, or the edges of the fistula sutured to the fistula base using a marsupialization technique with absorbable suture material. The wound usually heals in 4–6 weeks.

The objective of the *LIFT procedure* is to identify the intersphincteric tract of the fistula using a circumferential incision at the anal verge, excising and ligating the tract and excising or curetting the part of the tract from the external sphincter to the skin. This procedure preserves both sphincters.

It is best performed in the prone jackknife position.

Anatomical Points

The anus has two circular muscles, the internal sphincter (involuntary muscle) and the external sphincter (voluntary muscle) which control muscle tone and fecal/gas

Table 3.6 Laying open of anal fistula with/without excision (fistulotomy) estimated frequency of complications, risks, and consequences

Complications, risks, and consequences	Estimated frequency
Most significant/serious complications	
Infection[a] overall	0.1–1 %
Subcutaneous	0.1–1 %
Perianal abscess	0.1–1 %
Systemic sepsis[a]	0.1–1 %
Hepatic portal sepsis (rare)	0.1–1 %
Bleeding/hematoma formation[a]	1–5 %
Pain on passage of bowel actions[a]	50–80 %
Fecal incontinence	
Transient	1–5 %
Longer term/soiling (rare)	0.1–1 %
Recurrence of fistula(e)[a]	5–20 %
Rare significant/serious problems	
Missed pathology[a]	0.1–1 %
Chronic ulceration with hypergranulation[a]	0.1–1 %
Anal stenosis (rare)	<0.1 %
Multi-system failure (renal, pulmonary, cardiac failure)[a]	<0.1 %
Less serious complications	
Bruising	50–80 %
Residual pain/discomfort	
Short term (<4 weeks)	50–80 %
Longer term (>12 weeks)	0.1–1 %
Urinary retention/catheterization (males)	1–5 %
Scarring	0.1–1 %

[a]Dependent on underlying pathology, anatomy, surgical technique, and preferences

control, respectively. The anal cushions are transposed in the 3, 7, and 11 o'clock positions (12 o'clock being anterior) around the anus and carry blood vessels, which can become enlarged and engorged as hemorrhoidal tissue, which may render sphincterotomy difficult. Chronic scarring or perianal sepsis may also alter the anatomy.

Perspective

See Table 3.6. The long-term concern is incontinence because of the division of a significant length of external sphincter or internal sphincter. Rather than having absolute incontinence, the more common problem is urgent incontinence (fecal urgency), and this may be improved by pelvic floor exercises. Injury to the sphincter can be avoided by perioperative MRI scan, endorectal ultrasound, or clinical assessment over the degree of muscle at the time of fistulotomy. Should the surgeon be concerned, then either the LIFT procedure, advancement flap, or fibrin glue injection is recommended.

Bleeding is the most common immediate problem and this usually resolves spontaneously, although perianal bruising may be a problem and extensive submucosal bleeding may occasionally occur, but it is usually visible on clothing or toilet paper.

Local cellulitis and perianal abscess may occur primarily or secondary to a hematoma. Recurrent fistula and pain can be a problem. Incontinence, particularly incontinence for flatus can be a distressing initial symptom, but usually resolves. Incontinence for feces can occur usually resolving within weeks, but very rarely being permanent due to muscle division, denervation, and chronic scarring.

Major Complications

The main potential problem is **perianal pain**, which may be significant, especially on defecation after surgery, but usually settles within 5–7 days. **Incontinence** to flatus can occur, as can fecal incontinence, but this is very rare. Other complications are usually minor. Initial **bleeding** is usual after fistulotomy, but this usually settles quickly. Severe bleeding may occur but is very rare, although it may require **further surgery**. **Recurrent/persistent fistula**, **localized cellulitis**, and rarely **systemic infection** can occur.

Consent and Risk Reduction

Main Points to Explain

- Discomfort and pain
- Bleeding
- Problems with GA
- Recurrent fistula
- Fecal incontinence
- Infection
- Further surgery
- Risks without surgery

Seton Placement

Description

General anesthesia is usually used, but on occasions local anesthesia may be used. GA affords better examination of the anus and palpation of the sphincter muscles, particularly the internal sphincter.

The lithotomy or prone jackknife position is used, depending on the surgeon's preference. The prone jackknife position offers a better view of the anus for the operating surgeon and reduces the edema associated with the supine position, and any bleeding usually runs away from the operating surgeon into the rectum. Anesthetists sometimes object to the prone jackknife position, because of the physiological effects on the circulatory system and respiratory system. Views of the anal canal are greatly enhanced by the use of the operating anoscope such as the Fansler, Eisenhammer, or Parks anoscopes and the headlight.

There are five main types of fistulae: *submucosal* (superficial), *intersphincteric*, *transsphincteric*, *suprasphincteric*, and *extrasphincteric* (supralevator). Setons are often used for fistulae through or above the external sphincter that are at high risk of causing incontinence with fistulotomy.

The objective of this operation is to identify the anatomy of the fistula and insert a seton (heavy nylon, silk, or other nonabsorbable thread) through the fistula tract.

Goodsall's law dictates that a fistula tract with an external opening in the anterior half of the perianal region will usually open directly into the anal canal/rectum internally, whereas fistulae with an external opening in the posterior half of the perianal region will usually open into the posterior midline of the anal canal/rectum. A "holed" probe is gently passed along the fistula tract, the internal opening identified, and a seton placed through the open end of the probe. A soft, doubled vascular loop can be used as a seton and tied loosely.

The aim of the loose seton is to establish the anatomy of the fistula, allow adequate drainage, and, with the passage of time, lead to a more distal or superficial position of the fistula. This will often allow subsequent fistulotomy usually 4–8 weeks later with the incision of a minimal amount of sphincter.

Some surgeons prefer to use a tight seton and progressively tighten the seton that gradually transects the sphincter over several weeks.

Anatomical Points

The anus has two circular muscles, the internal sphincter (involuntary muscle) and the external sphincter (voluntary muscle) which control muscle tone and fecal/gas control, respectively. The anal cushions are transposed in the 3, 7, and 11 o'clock positions (12 o'clock being anterior) around the anus and carry blood vessels, which can become enlarged and engorged as hemorrhoidal tissue, which may render sphincterotomy difficult. Chronic scarring or perianal sepsis may also alter the anatomy.

Perspective

See Table 3.7. The aim of the seton is to avoid the long-term concern of incontinence arising from surgical laying open of a deep or high fistula due division of

Table 3.7 Seton placement estimated frequency of complications, risks, and consequences

Complications, risks, and consequences	Estimated frequency
Most significant/serious complications	
Infection[a] overall	0.1–1 %
Subcutaneous	0.1–1 %
Perianal abscess	0.1–1 %
Systemic sepsis[a]	0.1–1 %
Hepatic portal sepsis (rare)	0.1–1 %
Bleeding/hematoma formation[a]	1–5 %
Pain on passage of bowel actions[a]	50–80 %
Fecal incontinence	
Transient	1–5 %
Longer term/soiling (rare)	0.1–1 %
Creation of a false passage	1–5 %
Recurrence of fistula(e)[a]	5–20 %
Rare significant/serious problems	
Missed pathology[a]	0.1–1 %
Chronic ulceration with hypergranulation[a]	0.1–1 %
Anal stenosis (rare)	<0.1 %
Multi-system failure (renal, pulmonary, cardiac failure)[a]	<0.1 %
Less serious complications	
Bruising	50–80 %
Residual pain/discomfort	
Short term (<4 weeks)	50–80 %
Longer term (>12 weeks)	0.1–1 %
Urinary retention/catheterization (males)	1–5 %
Scarring	0.1–1 %

[a]Dependent on underlying pathology, anatomy, surgical technique, and preferences

the external sphincter. Some discomfort and minor incontinence can occur even with seton insertion, but this is usually well tolerated and relatively low grade.

Exploration of a complex deep fistula can result in inadvertent misplacement of the probe through the wall of the fistula tract making a false passage and perhaps complicating the fistula. A false internal opening can be inadvertently made in this way, and the seton may therefore be misplaced and less effective in treating the fistulous tract.

Bleeding is the most common immediate problem and this usually resolves spontaneously, although perianal bruising may be a problem and extensive submucosal bleeding may occasionally occur, but it is usually visible on clothing or toilet paper. Local cellulitis and perianal abscess may occur primarily or secondary to a hematoma. Recurrent fistula and pain can be a problem. Not making the seton too tight can reduce pain.

Incontinence, particularly incontinence for flatus can be a distressing initial symptom, but usually resolves. Incontinence for feces with simple seton insertion is very rare but can occur. A small amount of intermittent fecal leakage may occur especially with straining; purulent or feculent discharge may occur at other times.

The use of regular salt baths and a combined or a pad to the perineum may overcome the majority of their problem of pain and discharge. Forcing the probe through a fistulous tract may create a false passage and new fistula(e) that can worsen the outcome by making surgical treatment more complex and difficult. By using a blunt probe and passing it gently along the fistula while moving slightly side to side can usually safely follow the tract.

Major Complications

The main potential problems are **perianal pain**, which may be significant, especially on defecation after surgery, but usually settles within 5–7 days, and **persistent discharge** which may take 2–3 weeks to settle. **Incontinence** to flatus can occur, as can fecal incontinence, but this is very rare. **Inadvertent creation of a false passage** can be problematic with establishment of new openings, new fistulous tracts, delayed healing, and increased complexity. Other complications are usually minor. Initial **bleeding** is usual after seton insertion, but this usually settles quickly. Severe bleeding may occur but is very rare, although it may require **further surgery**. **Recurrent/persistent fistula**, **localized cellulitis**, and rarely **systemic infection** can occur. **Breakage of the seton** may require repeat insertion.

Consent and Risk Reduction

Main Points to Explain

- Discomfort and pain
- Bleeding
- Problems with GA
- Failure to cannulate the fistula
- Creation of a false passage
- Infection
- Fecal incontinence
- Breakage of seton
- Further surgery
- Risks without surgery

Mucosal Advancement Flap

Description

General anesthesia is usually used, but on occasions local anesthesia may be used. GA affords better examination of the anus and palpation of the sphincter muscles, particularly the internal sphincter.

The lithotomy or prone jackknife position is used, depending on the surgeon's preference. The prone jackknife position offers a better view of the anus for the operating surgeon and reduces the edema associated with the supine position, and any bleeding usually runs away from the operating surgeon into the rectum. Anesthetists sometimes object to the prone jackknife position, because of the physiological effects on the circulatory system and respiratory system. Views of the anal canal are greatly enhanced by the use of the operating anoscope such as the Fansler, Eisenhammer, or Parks anoscopes and a headlight.

There are five main types of fistulae: *submucosal* (superficial), *intersphincteric*, *transsphincteric*, *suprasphincteric*, and *extrasphincteric* (supralevator). Setons are often used for fistulae through or above the external sphincter that are at high risk of causing incontinence with fistulotomy.

The objective of the operation is to excise the external component of the fistula to the level of the external sphincter by "coring out" the external component using sharp dissection, and then the internal component of the fistula is excised including the internal opening and the internal sphincter component. A "U-" shaped flap of rectal mucosa is advanced to suture healthy mucosa over the excised internal opening of the fistula. Development of the flap is aided by submucosal injection of adrenaline solution and diathermy to reduce bleeding. The external wound is allowed to heal by secondary intention.

Anatomical Points

The anus has two circular muscles, the internal sphincter (involuntary muscle) and the external sphincter (voluntary muscle) which control muscle tone and fecal/gas control, respectively. The anal cushions are transposed in the 3, 7, and 11 o'clock positions (12 o'clock being anterior) around the anus and carry blood vessels, which can become enlarged and engorged as hemorrhoidal tissue, which may render sphincterotomy difficult. Chronic scarring or perianal sepsis may also alter the anatomy.

Perspective

See Table 3.8. Achieving a wide-based advancement flap is crucial to the success of the procedure to avoid flap necrosis. The flap should be 2 cm wider at its base than its apex to allow for a good blood supply at the base of the flap. Adequate access and illumination is vital. The use of the "lone star" retractor in the anus allows for better vision and eversion of the anoderm, and this is preferred by some surgeons for complex perianal procedures.

Flap necrosis, wound breakdown, and recurrent fistula are potential problems with anorectal flap repair. The long-term concern is incontinence because of the division of a significant length of external sphincter or internal sphincter.

Table 3.8 Mucosal advancement flap estimated frequency of complications, risks, and consequences

Complications, risks, and consequences	Estimated frequency
Most significant/serious complications	
Infection[a] overall	1–5 %
Subcutaneous	0.1–1 %
Perianal abscess	0.1–1 %
Systemic sepsis[a]	0.1–1 %
Hepatic portal sepsis (rare)	0.1–1 %
Bleeding/hematoma formation[a]	1–5 %
Pain on passage of bowel actions[a]	50–80 %
Fecal incontinence	
Transient	1–5 %
Longer term/soiling (rare)	0.1–1 %
Recurrence of fistula(e)[a]	1–5 %
Rare significant/serious problems	
Missed pathology[a]	0.1–1 %
Chronic ulceration with hypergranulation[a]	0.1–1 %
Flap necrosis	0.1–1 %
Anal stenosis (rare)	<0.1 %
Multi-system failure (renal, pulmonary, cardiac failure)[a]	<0.1 %
Less serious complications	
Bruising	50–80 %
Residual pain/discomfort	
Short term (<4 weeks)	50–80 %
Longer term (>12 weeks)	0.1–1 %
Urinary retention/catheterization (males)	1–5 %
Scarring	0.1–1 %

[a]Dependent on underlying pathology, anatomy, surgical technique, and preferences

Rather than having absolute incontinence, the more common problem is urgent incontinence (fecal urgency), and this may be improved by pelvic floor exercises. Injury to the sphincter can be avoided by perioperative MRI scan, endorectal ultrasound, or clinical assessment over the degree of muscle at the time of fistulotomy.

Bleeding is the most common immediate problem and this usually resolves spontaneously, although perianal bruising may be a problem and extensive submucosal bleeding may occasionally occur, but it is usually visible on clothing or toilet paper. Careful and gentle passage of a blunt probe may be helpful to define the fistula just before excision. Local cellulitis and perianal abscess may occur primarily or secondary to a hematoma.

Recurrent fistula, particularly in Crohn's disease, and pain can be a problem. Incontinence, particularly incontinence for flatus, can be a distressing initial symptom, but usually resolves. Incontinence for feces can occur usually resolving within weeks, but very rarely being permanent due to muscle division, denervation, and chronic scarring.

Major Complications

The main potential problem is **perianal pain**, which may be significant, especially on defecation after surgery, but usually settles within 5–7 days. **Flap necrosis, wound breakdown,** and **recurrent fistula** are potential problems with anorectal flap repair. **Incontinence** to flatus can occur, as can fecal incontinence, but this is uncommon. Other complications are usually minor. Initial **bleeding** is usual after fistula repair, but this usually settles quickly. Severe bleeding may occur but is very rare, although it may require **further surgery. Recurrent/persistent fistula, localized cellulitis**, and rarely **systemic infection** can occur.

Consent and Risk Reduction

Main Points to Explain

- Discomfort and pain
- Bleeding
- Problems with GA
- Failure to cannulate fistula
- Creation of a false tract
- Fecal incontinence
- Flap necrosis
- Infection
- Recurrent fistula(e)
- Further surgery
- Risks without surgery

Hemorrhoidectomy (Open or Stapled Techniques)

Description

General anesthesia is usually used, but on occasions local anesthesia may be used. GA affords better examination of the anus and palpation of the sphincter muscles, particularly the internal sphincter.

The lithotomy or prone jackknife position is used, depending on the surgeon's preference. The prone jackknife position offers a better view of the anus for the operating surgeon and reduces the edema associated with the supine position, and any bleeding usually runs away from the operating surgeon into the rectum. Anesthetists sometimes object to the prone jackknife position, because of the physiological effects on the circulatory system and respiratory system. Views of the anal canal are greatly enhanced by the use of the operating anoscope such as the Fansler, Eisenhammer, or Parks anoscopes and a headlight.

The indications for this surgery are those patients who have failed with or are unsuitable for conservative measures of high-fiber diet, injection sclerotherapy, or banding. Most patients have a significant external component (skin) as well as internal hemorrhoids.

The aim of *open hemorrhoidectomy* is to excise the hemorrhoidal tissue, including any external skin tag, together with ligation of the hemorrhoidal vessels, at the appropriate location(s) around the anus. The mucosa and skin at the edges of the defect can be left open or sutured. Only about 1/3 of the circumference of the anus should be excised to avoid anal stenosis.

The other surgical options are *stapled hemorrhoidectomy and transanal hemorrhoidal dearterialization (THD)*.

Anatomical Points

The anus has two circular muscles, the internal sphincter (involuntary muscle) and the external sphincter (voluntary muscle) which control muscle tone and fecal/gas control, respectively. The anal cushions are transposed in the 3, 7, and 11 o'clock positions (12 o'clock being anterior) around the anus and carry blood vessels, which can become enlarged and engorged as hemorrhoidal tissue, which may prolapse and extend externally. Chronic scarring, skin tags, or perianal sepsis may also alter the anatomy.

Perspective

See Table 3.9. The main complications are pain and bleeding. Bleeding is the most common immediate problem and this usually resolves spontaneously, and a small amount is almost usual, although perianal bruising may be a problem and extensive submucosal bleeding may occasionally occur, but it is usually visible on clothing or toilet paper. Infection is rare, but local cellulitis and perianal abscess can occur primarily or secondary to a hematoma. Pain with postoperative defecation is usual and typically settles over 5–7 days. Avoidance of constipation is paramount to avoiding severe pain. Pain can be reduced with good oral analgesia, laxatives, and lukewarm salt baths. Incontinence, particularly incontinence for flatus can be a distressing initial symptom, but usually resolves. Incontinence for feces is very uncommon but can occur usually resolving within weeks, but very rarely being permanent due to chronic scarring. Anal stenosis is a severe complication that should be avoidable with retention of the anal mucosa of >2/3 of the anal circumference. Stenosis is nearly always caused by the excessive excision of perianal skin and anoderm.

Table 3.9 Hemorrhoidectomy (open or stapled) estimated frequency of complications, risks, and consequences

Complications, risks, and consequences	Estimated frequency
Most significant/serious complications	
Bleeding/hematoma formation[a]	1–5 %
Pain on passage of bowel actions[a]	50–80 %
Fecal incontinence	
Transient	1–5 %
Longer term/soiling (rare)	0.1–1 %
Recurrence of hemorrhoids	5–20 %
Rare significant/serious problems	
Missed pathology[a]	0.1–1 %
Chronic ulceration with hypergranulation[a]	0.1–1 %
Discharge	
Anal stenosis (rare)	0.1–1 %
Infection[a] overall	0.1–1 %
Subcutaneous	0.1–1 %
Perianal abscess	0.1–1 %
Systemic sepsis[a]	0.1–1 %
Hepatic portal sepsis (rare)	0.1–1 %
Further surgery	0.1–1 %
Multi-system failure (renal, pulmonary, cardiac failure)[a]	<0.1 %
Less serious complications	
Bruising	50–80 %
Residual pain/discomfort	
Short term (<4 weeks)	50–80 %
Longer term (>12 weeks)	5–20 %
Urinary retention/catheterization (males)	1–5 %
Scarring	0.1–1 %

[a]Dependent on underlying pathology, anatomy, surgical technique, and preferences

Major Complications

The main potential problem is **perianal pain**, which may be significant, especially on defecation after surgery, but usually settles within 5–7 days. **Incontinence** to flatus can occur, as can fecal incontinence, but this is very rare. Other complications are usually minor. Initial **bleeding** is usual after hemorrhoidectomy, but this usually settles quickly. Severe bleeding may occur, particularly between 1 and 2 weeks postoperatively from a slipped pedicle ligature, but is rare, although it may require **further surgery**. **Recurrent/persistent hemorrhoids** are not uncommon, despite apparently adequate surgery. **Anal stenosis** is a severe complication that can usually be avoided by carefully leaving enough skin and mucosa, but if it occurs may require further surgery. Infection is very rare, but **localized cellulitis** and rarely **systemic infection** can occur.

Consent and Risk Reduction

Main Points to Explain

- Discomfort and pain
- Bleeding
- Problems with GA
- Infection
- Recurrent hemorrhoids
- Fecal incontinence
- Avoidance of constipation
- Anal stenosis
- Further surgery
- Risks without surgery

Further Reading, References, and Resources

Examination Under Anesthesia (+/– Anal Dilatation)

Billingham RP, Isler JT, Kimmins MH, Nelson JM, Schweitzer J, Murphy MM. The diagnosis and management of common anorectal disorders. Curr Probl Surg. 2004;41(7):586–645.

Perianal Abscess Drainage

Billingham RP, Isler JT, Kimmins MH, Nelson JM, Schweitzer J, Murphy MM. The diagnosis and management of common anorectal disorders. Curr Probl Surg. 2004;41(7):586–645.
Malik AI, Nelson RL. Surgical management of anal fistulae: a systematic review. Colorectal Dis. 2008;10:420–30.
Quah HM, Tang CL, Eu KW, Chan SYE, Samuel M. Meta-analysis of randomized clinical trials comparing drainage alone vs primary sphincter-cutting procedures for anorectal abscess–fistula. Int J Colorectal Dis. 2006;21:602–9.
Rickard MJFX. Review article: anal abscesses and fistulas. ANZ J Surg. 2005;75:64–72.

Ischiorectal Abscess Drainage

Billingham RP, Isler JT, Kimmins MH, Nelson JM, Schweitzer J, Murphy MM. The diagnosis and management of common anorectal disorders. Curr Probl Surg. 2004;41(7):586–645.
Malik AI, Nelson RL. Surgical management of anal fistulae: a systematic review. Colorectal Dis. 2008;10:420–30.

Quah HM, Tang CL, Eu KW, Chan SYE, Samuel M. Meta-analysis of randomized clinical trials comparing drainage alone vs primary sphincter-cutting procedures for anorectal abscess–fistula. Int J Colorectal Dis. 2006;21:602–9.
Rickard MJFX. Review article: anal abscesses and fistulas. ANZ J Surg. 2005;75:64–72.

Lateral Internal Sphincterotomy

Billingham RP, Isler JT, Kimmins MH, Nelson JM, Schweitzer J, Murphy MM. The diagnosis and management of common anorectal disorders. Curr Probl Surg. 2004;41(7):586–645.
Collins EE, Lund JN. A review of chronic anal fissure management. Tech Coloproctol. 2007;11: 209–23.

Anal Fissurectomy

Billingham RP, Isler JT, Kimmins MH, Nelson JM, Schweitzer J, Murphy MM. The diagnosis and management of common anorectal disorders. Curr Probl Surg. 2004;41(7):586–645.
Collins EE, Lund JN. A review of chronic anal fissure management. Tech Coloproctol. 2007;11: 209–23.

Laying Open of Anal Fistula with/Without Excision (Fistulotomy)

Billingham RP, Isler JT, Kimmins MH, Nelson JM, Schweitzer J, Murphy MM. The diagnosis and management of common anorectal disorders. Curr Probl Surg. 2004;41(7):586–645.
Malik AI, Nelson RL. Surgical management of anal fistulae: a systematic review. Colorectal Dis. 2008;10:420–30.
Quah HM, Tang CL, Eu KW, Chan SYE, Samuel M. Meta-analysis of randomized clinical trials comparing drainage alone vs primary sphincter-cutting procedures for anorectal abscess–fistula. Int J Colorectal Dis. 2006;21:602–9.
Rickard MJFX. Review article: anal abscesses and fistulas. ANZ J Surg. 2005;75:64–72.
Rojanasakul A. Total anal sphincter saving technique for fistula-in-ano. The ligation of the intersphincteric tract. J Med Assoc Thai. 2007;90:581–6.

Seton Placement

Billingham RP, Isler JT, Kimmins MH, Nelson JM, Schweitzer J, Murphy MM. The diagnosis and management of common anorectal disorders. Curr Probl Surg. 2004;41(7):586–645.
Malik AI, Nelson RL. Surgical management of anal fistulae: a systematic review. Colorectal Dis. 2008;10:420–30.

Quah HM, Tang CL, Eu KW, Chan SYE, Samuel M. Meta-analysis of randomized clinical trials comparing drainage alone vs primary sphincter-cutting procedures for anorectal abscess–fistula. Int J Colorectal Dis. 2006;21:602–9.

Rickard MJFX. Review article: anal abscesses and fistulas. ANZ J Surg. 2005;75:64–72.

Mucosal Advancement Flap

Billingham RP, Isler JT, Kimmins MH, Nelson JM, Schweitzer J, Murphy MM. The diagnosis and management of common anorectal disorders. Curr Probl Surg. 2004;41(7):586–645.

Malik AI, Nelson RL. Surgical management of anal fistulae: a systematic review. Colorectal Dis. 2008;10:420–30.

Quah HM, Tang CL, Eu KW, Chan SYE, Samuel M. Meta-analysis of randomized clinical trials comparing drainage alone vs primary sphincter-cutting procedures for anorectal abscess–fistula. Int J Colorectal Dis. 2006;21:602–9.

Rickard MJFX. Review article: anal abscesses and fistulas. ANZ J Surg. 2005;75:64–72.

Hemorrhoidectomy (Open or Stapled)

Billingham RP, Isler JT, Kimmins MH, Nelson JM, Schweitzer J, Murphy MM. The diagnosis and management of common anorectal disorders. Curr Probl Surg. 2004;41(7):586–645.

Collins EE, Lund JN. A review of chronic anal fissure management. Tech Coloproctol. 2007;11:209–23.

Dal Monte PP, Tagariello C, Giordano P. Transanal haemorrhoidal dearterialization: nonexcisional surgery for the treatment of haemorrhoidal disease. Tech Coloproctol. 2007;11:333–9.

Malik AI, Nelson RL. Surgical management of anal fistulae: a systematic review. Colorectal Dis. 2008;10:420–30.

Quah HM, Tang CL, Eu KW, Chan SYE, Samuel M. Meta-analysis of randomized clinical trials comparing drainage alone vs primary sphincter-cutting procedures for anorectal abscess–fistula. Int J Colorectal Dis. 2006;21:602–9.

Rickard MJFX. Review article: anal abscesses and fistulas. ANZ J Surg. 2005;75:64–72.

Shanmugam V, Thaha MA, Rabindranath KS, Campbell KL, Steele RJ, Loudon MA. Rubber band ligation versus excisional haemorrhoidectomy for haemorrhoids. Cochrane Database Syst Rev. 2005;20(3):CD005034.

Shanmugam V, Thaha MA, Rabindranath KS, Campbell KL, Steele RJ, Loudon MA. Systematic review of randomized trials comparing rubber band ligation with excisional haemorrhoidectomy. Br J Surg. 2005;92(12):1481–7.

Shao W-J, Li G-CH, Zhang ZH-K, Yang B-L, Sun G-D, Chen Y-Q. Systematic review and meta-analysis of randomized controlled trials comparing stapled haemorrhoidopexy with conventional haemorrhoidectomy. Br J Surg. 2008;95:147–60.

Sutherland LM, Burchard AK, Matsuda K, Sweeney JL, Bokey EL, Childs PA, Roberts AK, Waxman BP, Maddern GJ. A systematic review of stapled hemorrhoidectomy. Arch Surg. 2002;137:1395–406.

Chapter 4
Pilonidal Sinus Surgery

Bruce Waxman and Brendon J. Coventry

General Perspective and Overview

The relative risks and complications increase proportionately according to the type of procedure performed and the nature of the pathology or underlying disease process. When complex pilonidal sinus or abscess problems are present, the risks are usually increased. This is principally related to the surgical difficulty, ability to obtain adjacent unaffected healthy tissue, infection, hematoma formation, and ability to resect the disease. Risk of failure of direct wound closure is associated with infection, and this is often present preoperatively.

Resections for chronic sinuses and in the presence of established infection often carry higher risks associated with wound problems, including dehiscence and chronic wound dressings. Persistent infection, incomplete sinus/abscess resection, and immunosuppression add to the chronicity.

The main serious complication is **infection,** which can be minimized by the adequate mobilization, reduction of wound tension, and ensuring satisfactory blood supply. **Dehiscence** and **abscess formation** and even **systemic sepsis** can occur. **Multi-system failure** and **death** are very rare except in diabetics and immunosuppressed individuals. **Hematoma formation** may arise from oozing and this may predispose to infection. **Recurrence** is a significant issue, and further surgery is often warranted.

B. Waxman, BMedSc, MBBS, FRACS, FRCS(Eng), FACS
Academic Surgical Unit, Monash University, Monash Health
and Southern Clinical School, Dandenong, VIC, Australia

B.J. Coventry, BMBS, PhD, FRACS, FACS, FRSM (✉)
Discipline of Surgery, Royal Adelaide Hospital, University of Adelaide,
L5 Eleanor Harrald Building, North Terrace, 5000 Adelaide, SA, Australia
e-mail: brendon.coventry@adelaide.edu.au

B.J. Coventry (ed.), *Lower Abdominal and Perineal Surgery,*
Surgery: Complications, Risks and Consequences,
DOI 10.1007/978-1-4471-5469-3_4, © Springer-Verlag London 2014

Positioning on the operating table has been associated with increased risk of **deep venous thrombosis** and **nerve palsies**, especially in prolonged procedures.

Possible reduction in the risk of misunderstandings over complications or consequences from perineal surgery might be achieved by:
- Good explanation of the risks, aims, benefits, and limitations of the procedure(s)
- Useful planning considering the anatomy, approach, alternatives, and method
- Avoiding likely associated vessels and nerves
- Adequate clinical follow-up

With these factors and facts in mind, the information given in this chapter must be appropriately and discernibly interpreted and used.

Important Note

It should be emphasized that the risks and frequencies that are given here *represent derived figures*. These *figures are best estimates of relative frequencies across most institutions*, not merely the highest-performing ones, and as such are often representative of a number of studies, which include different patients with differing comorbidities and different surgeons. In addition, the risks of complications in lower- or higher-risk patients may lie outside these estimated ranges, and individual clinical judgment is required as to the expected risks communicated to the patient and staff or for other purposes. The range of risks is also derived from experience and the literature; while risks outside this range may exist, certain risks may be reduced or absent due to variations of procedures or surgical approaches. It is recognized that different patients, practitioners, institutions, regions, and countries may vary in their requirements and recommendations.

Pilonidal Abscess Incision and Drainage Surgery

Description

General anesthesia is usually used, but on occasions local anesthesia may be used. The aim of the procedure is to examine the natal cleft, pilonidal sinus(es), and pilonidal abscess, then drain the abscess or cyst using a cruciate incision, curette, lay-open the cavity, and pack with antiseptic gauze dressing, to settle the acute infection and pain. Adequate drainage is the main objective. GA affords better examination of the anus and palpation of the pilonidal cyst and is less painful. The prone jackknife or occasionally the lateral decubitus position can be used, depending on the surgeon's preference. The prone jackknife position offers a better view of the natal cleft for the operating surgeon, and any bleeding usually runs away from the operating surgeon. Anesthetists sometimes object to the prone jackknife position, because of the physiological effects on the circulatory system and respiratory system. Drainage alone often reduces the infection but seldom settles the pilonidal problem sufficiently, and persistent or recurrent symptoms are usual. Further definitive surgery may be necessary.

Anatomical Points

The natal cleft is a narrow moist region, often containing hair, which can develop cutaneous sinuses extending deep into the subcutaneous fat almost to the deep posterior sacral fascia. Hair (usually from the head) enters the sweat glands and forms cystic collections of keratin, sebum, and hair. Multiple sinuses are common, usually close to the midline. Induration and inflammation may distort the anatomy.

Perspective

See Table 4.1. Complications are usually of a minor nature but may be severe on occasions. Infection and inflammation are usually present as the main indication for surgical drainage. The main complications are infection, pain, and bleeding which are all extensions of the preoperative situation and dehiscence. Recurrence of the pilonidal sinus is very common after incision and drainage, since the underlying problem is often not alleviated.

Table 4.1 Pilonidal abscess incision and drainage estimated frequency of complications, risks, and consequences

Complications, risks, and consequences	Estimated frequency
Most significant/serious complications	
Infection[a] overall	1–5 %
Subcutaneous	1–5 %
Systemic sepsis[a]	0.1–1 %
Recurrence of pilonidal sinus[a]	5–20 %
Chronic discharge	5–20 %
Further surgery	5–20 %
Dehiscence and chronic wound dressings	50–80 %
Rare significant/serious problems	
Bleeding/hematoma formation[a]	
Wound (immediate or delayed)	0.1–1 %
Missed pathology[a]	0.1–1 %
Chronic ulceration with hypergranulation[a]	0.1–1 %
Less serious complications	
Residual pain/discomfort/tenderness	
Short term (<4 weeks)	50–80 %
Longer term (>12 weeks) soiling	0.1–1 %
Scarring	0.1–1 %
Urinary retention/catheterization (males)	1–5 %

[a]Dependent on underlying pathology, anatomy, surgical technique, and preferences

Major Complications

The main complication is **pain**, which is often adequately controlled with oral analgesia. Pain with **dehiscence** (or open management) and **chronic dressings** is also common. **Purulent discharge** is not uncommon, but usually settles with repeated dressings. **Bleeding** is not uncommon, but is rarely great in volume. **Infection** is usually present before surgery, as is some element of surrounding **cellulitis**, but on occasions these can worsen. **Systemic sepsis** is very rare but can occur. **Further surgery** is usual after simple drainage. **Urinary retention and catheterization** are not uncommon in males with any form of perineal or groin surgery. **Recurrence** is not uncommon and often requires **further surgery**.

Consent and Risk Reduction

Main Points to Explain

- Discomfort/pain
- Infection
- Recurrence
- Bleeding
- Delayed healing
- Chronic dressings
- Further surgery

Pilonidal Sinus Excision and Laying Open

Description

General anesthesia is usually used, but on occasions local anesthesia may be used. GA affords better examination of the anus and palpation of the pilonidal cyst and is less painful. The prone jackknife or occasionally the lateral decubitus position can be used, depending on the surgeon's preference. The prone jackknife position offers a better view of the natal cleft for the operating surgeon, and any bleeding usually runs away from the operating surgeon. Anesthetists sometimes object to the prone jackknife position, because of the physiological effects on the circulatory system and respiratory system.

The aim of the procedure is to examine the natal cleft, pilonidal sinus(es), and pilonidal abscess, then excise the pilonidal sinuses and cyst using an elliptical excision, and then pack the cavity with antiseptic gauze, alginate, or occasionally vacuum-assisted dressings. Complete removal of the sinus tracts is the main objective. The other option is marsupialization of the skin edges to the base of the wound.

Anatomical Points

The natal cleft is a narrow moist region, often containing hair, which can develop cutaneous sinuses extending deep into the subcutaneous fat almost to the deep posterior sacral fascia. Hair (usually from the head) enters the sweat glands and forms cystic collections of keratin, sebum, and hair. Multiple sinuses are common, usually close to the midline. Induration and inflammation may distort the anatomy. The pilonidal cyst may be midline or eccentric.

Perspective

See Table 4.2. Complications are usually of a minor nature but may be severe on occasions. Infection and inflammation may be present to some degree. The main complications are infection, pain, and bleeding which are all extensions of the low-grade preoperative situation. Recurrence of the sinuses and cyst can occur after excision.

Table 4.2 Pilonidal sinus excision and laying open estimated frequency of complications, risks, and consequences

Complications, risks, and consequences	Estimated frequency
Most significant/serious complications	
Infection[a] overall	1–5 %
Subcutaneous	1–5 %
Systemic sepsis[a]	0.1–1 %
Recurrence of pilonidal sinus[a]	5–20 %
Chronic discharge	5–20 %
Further surgery	5–20 %
Chronic wound dressings	80 %
Rare significant/serious problems	
Bleeding/hematoma formation[a]	
Wound (immediate or delayed)	0.1–1 %
Missed pathology[a]	0.1–1 %
Chronic ulceration with hypergranulation[a]	0.1–1 %
Less serious complications	
Residual pain/discomfort/tenderness	
Short term (<4 weeks)	50–80 %
Longer term (>12 weeks) soiling	0.1–1 %
Scarring	0.1–1 %
Urinary retention/catheterization (males)	1–5 %

[a]Dependent on underlying pathology, anatomy, surgical technique, and preferences

Major Complications

The main complication is **pain**, which is often adequately controlled with oral analgesia. Pain with the **chronic dressings** is also common. **Purulent discharge** is not uncommon, but usually settles with repeated dressings. **Bleeding** is not uncommon, but is rarely great in volume. **Infection** is usually present before surgery, as is some element of surrounding **cellulitis**, but on occasions these can worsen. **Systemic sepsis** is very rare but can occur. **Urinary retention and catheterization** are not uncommon in males with any form of perineal or groin surgery. **Recurrence** is not uncommon and often requires **further surgery**.

Consent and Risk Reduction

Main Points to Explain

- Discomfort/pain
- Infection
- Recurrence
- Bleeding
- Delayed healing
- Chronic dressings
- Further surgery

Pilonidal Sinus Excision and Primary Closure/ Flap Repair (Karydakis Procedure)

Description

General anesthesia is usually used, but on occasions local anesthesia may be used. GA affords better examination of the anus and palpation of the pilonidal cyst and is less painful. The prone jackknife or occasionally the lateral decubitus position can be used, depending on the surgeon's preference. The prone jackknife position offers a better view of the natal cleft for the operating surgeon, and any bleeding usually runs away from the operating surgeon. Anesthetists sometimes object to the prone jackknife position, because of the physiological effects on the circulatory system and respiratory system.

The aim of the procedure is to examine the natal cleft, pilonidal sinus(es), and pilonidal abscess, excise the pilonidal sinuses and cyst completely, and then close the defect. A rotation flap can be used to fill the defect. Complete excision is the main objective. The Karydakis method is an unequal elliptical excision, undermining one edge to create a local rotation flap which when closed moves the natal cleft and the wound laterally, reducing the depth of the cleft considerably and reducing risk of recurrence. Alternatively, a rhomboidal or other rotation flap repair or V-Y advancement flap can be used to fill the defect after pilonidal sinus/cyst excision.

Anatomical Points

The natal cleft is a narrow moist region, often containing hair, which can develop cutaneous sinuses extending deep into the subcutaneous fat almost to the deep posterior sacral fascia. Hair (usually from the head) enters the glands and forms cystic collections of keratin, sebum, and hair. Multiple sinuses are common, usually close to the midline. Induration and inflammation may distort the anatomy.

Perspective

See Table 4.3. Complications are usually of a minor nature but may be severe on occasions. Infection and inflammation may be present at low levels preoperatively. The main complications are infection, pain, and bleeding which are all extensions

Table 4.3 Pilonidal sinus excision and primary or flap closure estimated frequency of complications, risks, and consequences

Complications, risks, and consequences	Estimated frequency
Most significant/serious complications	
Infection[a] overall	1–5 %
Subcutaneous	1–5 %
Systemic sepsis[a]	0.1–1 %
Bleeding/hematoma formation[a]	1–5 %
Wound (immediate or delayed)	
Wound breakdown/dehiscence	1–5 %
Flap necrosis	1–5 %
Recurrence of pilonidal sinus[a]	5–20 %
Chronic discharge	5–20 %
Further surgery	5–20 %
Rare significant/serious problems	
Missed pathology[a]	0.1–1 %
Chronic ulceration with hypergranulation[a]	0.1–1 %
Less serious complications	
Residual pain/discomfort	
Short term (<4 weeks)	50–80 %
Longer term (>12 weeks) soiling	0.1–1 %
Scarring/poor cosmesis	0.1–1 %
Chronic wound dressings	1–5 %
Urinary retention/catheterization (males)	1–5 %

[a]Dependent on underlying pathology, anatomy, surgical technique, and preferences

of the preoperative situation. Recurrence of the sinuses and cyst can occur after excision and repair.

Major Complications

The main complication is **pain**, which is often adequately controlled with oral analgesia. **Hemoserous discharge** is not uncommon, but usually settles with repeated dressings. **Bleeding** is not uncommon, but is rarely great in volume. **Infection** is usually present to some degree before surgery, as is some element of surrounding **cellulitis**, but on occasions these can worsen and may be followed by **dehiscence**. **Systemic sepsis** is very rare but can occur. **Flap necrosis** can occur where this method is used for repair of the defect and can contribute to dehiscence. **Urinary retention and catheterization** are not uncommon in males with any form of perineal or groin surgery. **Recurrence** is not uncommon and often requires **further surgery**.

Consent and Risk Reduction

Main Points to Explain

- Discomfort/pain
- Infection
- Recurrence
- Bleeding
- Delayed healing
- Flap/wound dehiscence
- Chronic dressings
- Further surgery

Further Reading, References, and Resources

Akin M, Gokbayir H, Kilic K, Topgul K, Ozdemir E, Ferahkose Z. Rhomboid excision and Limberg flap for managing pilonidal sinus: long-term results in 411 patients. Colorectal Dis. 2008;10(9):945–8.

Bascom J, Bascom T. Prevention of wound healing disorders and recurrence. Am J Surg. 2009;198(2):293–4.

Can MF, Sevinc MM, Yilmaz M. Comparison of Karydakis flap reconstruction versus primary midline closure in sacrococcygeal pilonidal disease: results of 200 military service members. Surg Today. 2009;39(7):580–6.

Carriquiry LA. Outcome of the rhomboid flap for recurrent pilonidal disease. World J Surg. 2009;33(5):1069.

Clemente CD. Anatomy – a regional atlas of the human body. 4th ed. Baltimore: Williams and Wilkins; 1997.

Doll D. Sinotomy versus excisional surgery for pilonidal sinus. ANZ J Surg. 2007;77(7):599–600. Author reply 600.

Doll D, Matevossian E, Wietelmann K, Evers T, Kriner M, Petersen S. Family history of pilonidal sinus predisposes to earlier onset of disease and a 50 % long-term recurrence rate. Dis Colon Rectum. 2009;52(9):1610–5.

el-Khadrawy O, Hashish M, Ismail K, Shalaby H. Outcome of the rhomboid flap for recurrent pilonidal disease. World J Surg. 2009;33(5):1064–8.

Jamieson GG. The anatomy of general surgical operations. 2nd ed. Edinburgh: Churchill Livingston; 2006.

Karakayali F, Karagulle E, Karabulut Z, Oksuc E, Moray G, Haberal M. Unroofing and marsupialization vs. rhomboid excision and Limberg flap in pilonidal disease: a prospective, randomized, clinical trial. Dis Colon Rectum. 2009;52(3):496–502.

Keshava A, Young CJ, Rickard MJ, Sinclair G. Karydakis flap repair for sacrococcygeal pilonidal sinus disease: how important is technique? ANZ J Surg. 2007;77(3):181–3.

Kitchen P. Pilonidal sinus: has off-midline closure become the gold standard? ANZ J Surg. 2009;79(1–2):4–5.

Mahdy T. Surgical treatment of the pilonidal disease: primary closure or flap reconstruction after excision. Dis Colon Rectum. 2008;51(12):1816–22.

McCallum IJ, King PM, Bruce J. Healing by primary closure versus open healing after surgery for pilonidal sinus: systematic review and meta-analysis. BMJ. 2008;336(7649):868–71. Review.

Mentes O, Oysul A, Harlak A, Zeybek N, Kozak O, Tufan T. Ultrasonography accurately evaluates the dimension and shape of the pilonidal sinus. Clinics (Sao Paulo). 2009;64(3):189–92.

Nursal TZ, Ezer A, Calişkan K, Törer N, Belli S, Moray G. Prospective randomized controlled trial comparing V-Y advancement flap with primary suture methods in pilonidal disease. Am J Surg. 2010;199(2):170–7.

Stewart A, Donoghue J, Mitten-Lewis S. Pilonidal sinus: healing rates, pain and embarrassment levels. J Wound Care. 2008;17(11):468–70. 472, 474.

Toccaceli S, Persico Stella L, Diana M, Dandolo R, Negro P. Treatment of pilonidal sinus with primary closure. A twenty-year experience. Chir Ital. 2008;60(3):433–8.

Winter D. Perspectives on vacuum-assisted closure therapy in pilonidal sinus surgery. Dis Colon Rectum. 2005;48(9):1829. Author reply 1829–30.

Chapter 5
Penile, Scrotal, and Testicular Surgery

Brendon J. Coventry and Villis Marshall

General Perspective and Overview

The relative risks and complications increase proportionately according to the type of procedure performed and the nature of the pathology or underlying disease process. When complex problems are present, the risks are usually increased. This is principally related to the surgical difficulty, ability to obtain adjacent unaffected healthy tissue, infection, hematoma formation, and ability to resect the disease. Risk of failure of direct wound closure is associated with infection, and this is often present preoperatively.

The main serious complication is **infection,** which can be minimized by the adequate mobilization, reduction of wound tension, and ensuring satisfactory blood supply. **Dehiscence** and **abscess formation** and even **systemic sepsis** can occur. **Multi-system failure** and **death** are very rare except in diabetics and immunosuppressed individuals. **Hematoma formation** may arise from oozing and this may predispose to infection. **Recurrence** is a significant issue, and further surgery is often warranted.

Positioning on the operating table has been associated with increased risk of **deep venous thrombosis** and **nerve palsies,** especially in prolonged procedures.

Possible reduction in the risk of misunderstandings over complications or consequences from penile, scrotal, or testicular surgery might be achieved by:

- Good explanation of the risks, aims, benefits, and limitations of the procedure(s)
- Useful planning considering the anatomy, approach, alternatives, and method

B.J. Coventry, BMBS, PhD, FRACS, FACS, FRSM (✉)
Discipline of Surgery, Royal Adelaide Hospital, University of Adelaide,
L5 Eleanor Harrald Building, North Terrace, 5000 Adelaide, SA, Australia
e-mail: brendon.coventry@adelaide.edu.au

V. Marshall, MD, FRACS
Royal Adelaide Hospital, University of Adelaide,
L5 Eleanor Harrald Building, North Terrace, 5000 Adelaide, SA, Australia

B.J. Coventry (ed.), *Lower Abdominal and Perineal Surgery,*
Surgery: Complications, Risks and Consequences,
DOI 10.1007/978-1-4471-5469-3_5, © Springer-Verlag London 2014

- Avoiding likely associated vessels and nerves
- Adequate clinical follow-up

With these factors and facts in mind, the information given in this chapter must be appropriately and discernibly interpreted and used.

Important Note
It should be emphasized that the risks and frequencies that are given here *represent derived figures*. These *figures are best estimates of relative frequencies across most institutions*, not merely the highest-performing ones, and as such are often representative of a number of studies, which include different patients with differing comorbidities and different surgeons. In addition, the risks of complications in lower- or higher-risk patients may lie outside these estimated ranges, and individual clinical judgment is required as to the expected risks communicated to the patient and staff or for other purposes. The range of risks is also derived from experience and the literature; while risks outside this range may exist, certain risks may be reduced or absent due to variations of procedures or surgical approaches. It is recognized that different patients, practitioners, institutions, regions, and countries may vary in their requirements and recommendations.

Circumcision

Description

General anesthetic is usually used for adults and children, but when small infants are circumcised using a plastic ring device, local anesthetic cream may be used, or occasionally no anesthesia may be required. Spinal anesthesia may be used on occasions. The aim is to remove the foreskin proximally to behind the glans penis. This exposes the glans permanently. The medical indications for circumcision are severe phimosis (stenosis), recurrent infections (with or without meatal stenosis), and recurrent paraphimosis. Acute severe paraphimosis is sometimes treated with hyaluronidase injections with reduction or a dorsal slit through the constricting band.

Anatomical Points

The foreskin ranges from minimal to very redundant, and physiological adhesions may join the penis to the foreskin in some people.

Table 5.1 Circumcision estimated frequency of complications, risks, and consequences

Complications, risks, and consequences	Estimated frequency
Most significant/serious complications	
Infection[a] overall	1–5 %
Subcutaneous	1–5 %
Systemic sepsis[a]	<0.1 %
Penile swelling	50–80 %
Rare significant/serious problems	
Bleeding/hematoma formation[a]	
Wound (immediate or delayed)	0.1–1 %
Wound breakdown/dehiscence	0.1–1 %
Chronic ulceration with hypergranulation[a]	0.1–1 %
Sensory changes	0.1–1 %
Chronic discharge	0.1–1 %
Meatal ulceration/stenosis	0.1–1 %
Paraphimosis (contraction band formation)	0.1–1 %
Phimosis (excess loose foreskin)	0.1–1 %
Excessive removal of foreskin	0.1–1 %
Further surgery (revision or hematoma drainage)	0.1–1 %
Less serious complications	
Residual pain/discomfort/tenderness	
Short term (<4 weeks)	50–80 %
Longer term (>12 weeks)	0.1–1 %
Chronic wound dressings	0.1–1 %
Urinary retention/catheterization	0.1–1 %
Scarring/poor cosmesis	0.1–1 %

[a]Dependent on underlying pathology, anatomy, surgical technique, and preferences

Perspective

See Table 5.1. Complications are generally minor and infrequent; however, some may be more significant on occasions. These include infection, skin necrosis, cosmetic deformity, removing too much or too little skin, meatal ulceration, meatal stenosis, and bleeding. Urinary retention is not uncommon and occasionally requires catheterization. Painful bandages especially with erection can be severe and require loosening and re-bandaging. Cosmetic deformity, although medically less serious, can be significant and serious to the patient, especially if the indication is for social or cosmetic reasons. Mortality is reported but extremely rare.

Major Complications

Pain may be significant and may require loosening of dressings and pain relief. **Bleeding** is rarely severe. **Infection** usually responds to local dressings and oral antibiotics if required. Infection may increase **scarring** and create **poor cosmesis**. **Meatal ulceration** may lead to **meatal stenosis** on occasions, which rarely can require further surgery. **Systemic sepsis** is very rare but can occur. **Wound necrosis** can occur and can contribute to dehiscence. **Further surgery** may be required. **Urinary retention and catheterization** are not uncommon in older males with any form of perineal or groin surgery. **Cosmetic deformity**, especially after infection, may be significant.

Consent and Risk Reduction

Main Points to Explain

- Discomfort/pain
- Infection
- Bleeding
- Meatal ulceration
- Meatal stenosis
- Delayed healing
- Flap/wound dehiscence
- Chronic dressings
- Cosmetic deformity
- Further surgery

Surgery for Meatal Stenosis

Description

General anesthetic is usually used for adults and children. Spinal anesthesia may be used on occasions. The aim is to dilate the closed urethral opening, and often a small incision is necessary. Rarely, a transposition skin/mucosal flap repair is required, often as a secondary procedure after simple surgery has failed.

Anatomical Points

The associated anatomy is relatively constant, but the degree of stenosis can vary considerably from mild narrowing altering the urine stream to complete closure. The presence of the foreskin can make the procedure more difficult, especially if phimosis is present.

Table 5.2 Surgery for meatal stenosis estimated frequency of complications, risks, and consequences

Complications, risks, and consequences	Estimated frequency
Most significant/serious complications	
Infection[a] overall	1–5 %
Subcutaneous	1–5 %
Urinary	1–5 %
Systemic sepsis[a]	<0.1 %
Penile swelling	50–80 %
Meatal ulceration/restenosis	1–5 %
Rare significant/serious problems	
Bleeding/hematoma formation[a]	
Wound (immediate or delayed)	0.1–1 %
Wound breakdown/dehiscence	0.1–1 %
Paraphimosis (contraction band formation)[a]	0.1–1 %
Phimosis (excess loose foreskin)[a]	0.1–1 %
Chronic ulceration with hypergranulation[a]	0.1–1 %
Sensory changes	0.1–1 %
Chronic discharge	0.1–1 %
Further surgery (revision or hematoma drainage)	1–5 %
Less serious complications	
Residual pain/discomfort/tenderness	
Short term (<4 weeks)	50–80 %
Longer term (>12 weeks)	0.1–1 %
Chronic wound dressings	0.1–1 %
Urinary retention/catheterization	0.1–1 %
Scarring/poor cosmesis	0.1–1 %

[a]Dependent on underlying pathology, anatomy, surgical technique, and preferences

Perspective

See Table 5.2. Complications are generally minor and/or infrequent; however, some may be more significant on occasions. These include infection, skin necrosis, cosmetic deformity, meatal ulceration, meatal restenosis, and bleeding. Urinary retention is not uncommon and occasionally requires catheterization. Acute dysuria is a typical feature until the skin and mucosa heal.

Major Complications

Pain may be significant and may require loosening of dressings and pain relief. **Acute dysuria** is a consequence of surgery and expected; if prolonged beyond 72 h, it is abnormal. **Bleeding** is rarely severe. **Infection** usually responds to local dressings and oral antibiotics, if required. Infection may increase **scarring** and create **poor cosmesis**. **Meatal ulceration** may lead to **recurrent meatal stenosis** on occasions, which may require further surgery.

Consent and Risk Reduction

Main Points to Explain

- Discomfort/pain
- Infection
- Bleeding
- Meatal ulceration
- Meatal restenosis
- Delayed healing
- Wound dehiscence
- Chronic dressings
- Cosmetic deformity
- Further surgery

Bilateral Fixation of Testes/Exploration of the Testes (Testicular Torsion)

Description

General anesthetic is almost always used; however, spinal anesthesia may be used. The aim is to explore the scrotal contents in particular the testes, as the usual indication for bilateral fixation is proven or suspected torsion of one testis. A separate transverse scrotal incision for each side, or a single midline incision, through the layers of the scrotum, may be used to expose each testis and deliver it outside the scrotum for adequate inspection. The color of the testis is noted and any evidence of torsion. If the testis is black or dark, then a period of time is spent waiting for any color change. Most testes will gain a pink coloration; however, if established necrosis has occurred (~>6 h ischemia time), then removal of the testis may be required. The procedure objective of detorsion and fixation to prevent future torsion is achieved by one of several methods, all of which fixate each testis to the scrotal median raphe or to the lateral scrotal tissues or both and sometimes to each other. Either absorbable or nonabsorbable sutures can be used.

Anatomical Points

The main cause for testicular torsion is high investment of the processus vaginalis around the testis and posterior epididymis, allowing the testis and epididymis to rotate

Table 5.3 Bilateral fixation of testes/exploration of the testes estimated frequency of complications, risks, and consequences

Complications, risks, and consequences	Estimated frequency
Most significant/serious complications	
Infection[a] overall	1–5 %
Subcutaneous	1–5 %
Systemic sepsis[a]	<0.1 %
Scrotal swelling	50–80 %
Rare significant/serious problems	
Bleeding/hematoma formation (scrotal)[a]	
Wound (immediate or delayed)	0.1–1 %
Wound breakdown/dehiscence	0.1–1 %
Wound sinus/suture granuloma	0.1–1 %
Further surgery (revision or hematoma drainage)	0.1–1 %
Chronic discharge	<0.1 %
Recurrent torsion	<0.1 %
Less serious complications	
Residual pain/discomfort/tenderness	
Short term (<4 weeks)	50–80 %
Longer term (>12 weeks)	0.1–1 %
Sensory changes	<0.1 %
Urinary retention/catheterization	0.1–1 %
Scarring/poor cosmesis	<0.1 %

[a]Dependent on underlying pathology, anatomy, surgical technique, and preferences

around the spermatic cord superiorly. This often produces the clinical "bell clapper" testis phenomenon, with a classical horizontal lie of the testis. Tenderness over the upper epididymis may signify torsion of an appendix of the testis; however, surgical exploration is usually warranted to confirm this, although duplex ultrasound can be very reliable in determining blood supply to each testis and the correct diagnosis.

Perspective

See Table 5.3. Complications are generally minor; however, on occasions some may be more significant. These include bleeding, hematoma formation, infection, skin necrosis, wound dehiscence, cosmetic deformity, acute and chronic pain, and rarely recurrent torsion. Urinary retention is not uncommon and occasionally requires catheterization. Large scrotal hematomas or infection can significantly increase hospitalization and delay recovery.

Major Complications

Pain may be significant and may require support dressings and pain relief. Chronic pain occasionally occurs and is a major problem. **Bleeding** is rarely severe but can produce a large scrotal hematoma requiring surgical evacuation. **Infection** usually responds to local dressings and oral antibiotics. Infection may cause wound dehiscence, increase **scarring,** and create **poor cosmesis**.

Consent and Risk Reduction

Main Points to Explain

- Discomfort/pain
- Infection
- Bleeding
- Delayed healing
- Wound dehiscence
- Recurrent torsion
- Cosmetic deformity
- Further surgery

Hydrocele Repair

Description

General anesthesia is almost always used; however, spinal anesthesia may be used. The aim is to explore the scrotal contents on the side of the hydrocele, confirm the diagnosis, and incise, drain, and repair the hydrocele. A separate transverse scrotal incision on the affected side, or a single midline incision, through the layers of the scrotum, is used, to expose the hydrocele. Several methods can be used to drain the hydrocele and prevent recurrence. A standard method excises some of the anterior part of the hydrocele sac and folds the lateral part of the hydrocele wall back against the epididymis where it is sutured with a continuous absorbable suture (Jaboulay method), on each side of the testis. This effectively obliterates the tunica vaginalis preventing reformation of the hydrocele. The scrotum is closed in layers. The procedure is usually unilateral, unless both sides are affected. Needle aspiration or tapping of the hydrocele is usually associated with recurrence.

Anatomical Points

The main cause for hydrocele is collection of excessive fluid in the tunica vaginalis, the remnant of the embryological processus vaginalis around the testis and posterior epididymis. A hydrocele invests the testis, predominantly anteriorly as a uniform

Table 5.4 Hydrocele repair estimated frequency of complications, risks, and consequences

Complications, risks, and consequences	Estimated frequency
Most significant/serious complications	
Infection[a] overall	1–5 %
Subcutaneous	1–5 %
Systemic sepsis[a]	<0.1 %
Scrotal swelling	50–80 %
Rare significant/serious problems	
Bleeding/hematoma formation (scrotal)[a]	
Wound (immediate or delayed)	0.1–1 %
Wound breakdown/dehiscence	0.1–1 %
Reformation of hydrocele	0.1–1 %
Wound sinus/suture granuloma	0.1–1 %
Further surgery (revision or hematoma drainage)	0.1–1 %
Less serious complications	
Residual pain/discomfort/tenderness	
Short term (<4 weeks)	50–80 %
Longer term (>12 weeks)	0.1–1 %
Sensory changes	<0.1 %
Chronic discharge	<0.1 %
Urinary retention/catheterization	0.1–1 %
Scarring/poor cosmesis	<0.1 %

[a]Dependent on underlying pathology, anatomy, surgical technique, and preferences

swelling, with the epididymis usually being palpable at the back. Duplex ultrasound can be very reliable in determining the correct diagnosis.

Perspective

See Table 5.4. Complications are generally minor; however, on occasions some may be more significant. These include bleeding, hematoma formation, infection, skin necrosis, wound dehiscence, cosmetic deformity, acute and chronic pain, and rarely recurrent hydrocele. Urinary retention is not uncommon and occasionally requires catheterization. Needle aspiration or tapping of the hydrocele is usually associated with recurrence, bleeding, and infection.

Major Complications

Pain may be significant and may require support dressings and pain relief. Chronic pain occasionally occurs and is a major problem. **Bleeding** is rarely severe but can produce a large hematoma requiring surgical evacuation. **Infection** usually responds to local dressings and oral antibiotics. Infection may cause wound dehiscence, increase **scarring,** and create **poor cosmesis**. **Recurrence** of the hydrocele may also occur, perhaps necessitating further surgery.

Consent and Risk Reduction

Main Points to Explain

- Discomfort/pain
- Infection
- Bleeding
- Delayed healing
- Wound dehiscence
- Recurrent hydrocele
- Cosmetic deformity
- Further surgery

Epididymal Cyst Resection

Description

General anesthesia is almost always used; however, spinal anesthesia may be used. The aim is to explore the scrotal contents on the side of the epididymal cyst, confirm the diagnosis, and excise and repair the epididymal cyst. A separate transverse scrotal incision on the affected side, or a single midline incision, through the layers of the scrotum, is used, to expose the epididymal cyst(s). Several methods can be used to excise the epididymal cyst and prevent recurrence. A standard method excises epididymal cyst and sutures the cyst opening against the epididymis with an absorbable suture. This effectively removes the epididymal cyst. The scrotum is closed in layers. The procedure is usually unilateral, unless both sides are symptomatic, although both sides are usually affected.

Anatomical Points

The main cause for an epididymal cyst is collection of excessive fluid in an embryological remnant at the superior pole of the epididymis, slightly posteriorly to the testis. Epididymal cysts are usually bilateral, being also palpable at the posterior-superior aspect of the epididymis. Duplex ultrasound can be very reliable in determining the correct diagnosis.

Table 5.5 Epididymal cyst resection estimated frequency of complications, risks, and consequences

Complications, risks, and consequences	Estimated frequency
Most significant/serious complications	
Infection[a] overall	1–5 %
Subcutaneous	1–5 %
Systemic sepsis[a]	<0.1 %
Scrotal swelling[a]	50–80 %
Rare significant/serious problems	
Bleeding/hematoma formation (scrotal)[a]	
Wound (immediate or delayed)	0.1–1 %
Wound breakdown/dehiscence	0.1–1 %
Reformation of epididymal cyst[a]	0.1–1 %
Infertility[a]	0.1–1 %
Wound sinus/suture granuloma	0.1–1 %
Sensory changes	<0.1 %
Chronic discharge	<0.1 %
Further surgery (revision or hematoma drainage)	0.1–1 %
Less serious complications	
Residual pain/discomfort/tenderness	
Short term (<4 weeks)	50–80 %
Longer term (>12 weeks)	0.1–1 %
Urinary retention/catheterization	0.1–1 %
Scarring/poor cosmesis	<0.1 %

[a]Dependent on underlying pathology, anatomy, surgical technique, and preferences

Perspective

See Table 5.5. Complications are generally minor; however, on occasions some may be more significant. These include bleeding, hematoma formation, infection, skin necrosis, wound dehiscence, cosmetic deformity, acute and chronic pain, and rarely recurrent epididymal cysts. Urinary retention is not uncommon and occasionally requires catheterization. A potentially serious complication is infertility due to scarring in the surgically operated testis, which may be significant if the other testis is also infertile and if fertility is desired.

Major Complications

Pain may be significant and may require support dressings and pain relief. Chronic pain occasionally occurs and is a major problem. **Bleeding** is rarely severe but can produce a large hematoma requiring surgical evacuation. **Infection** usually responds to local dressings and oral antibiotics. Infection may cause wound dehiscence, increase **scarring,** and create **poor cosmesis**. **Infertility** may occur and may be significant in a male desiring fertility. **Recurrence** of the epididymal cyst is also possible. Infertility is a possible problem for men desiring childbearing ability.

Consent and Risk Reduction

Main Points to Explain

- Discomfort/pain
- Infection
- Bleeding
- Delayed healing
- Wound dehiscence
- Recurrent cyst
- Infertility
- Cosmetic deformity
- Further surgery

Orchidectomy

Description

General anesthesia is almost always used; however, spinal anesthesia may be used. The aim of bilateral orchidectomy is to gain the scrotal contents on each side, suture-ligate the spermatic cord with a heavy absorbable suture, and excise the testes and epididymis. A separate transverse scrotal incision on each side, or a single midline incision, through the layers of the scrotum, is used, to expose the testes. This effectively removes both testes, usually indicated for removal of testosterone for treatment of metastatic prostate cancer. The scrotum is closed in layers. The need for this procedure has declined with the advent of the raft of testosterone inhibitors and blockers. Unilateral orchidectomy for testicular carcinoma or other tumors is usually performed through an ipsilateral groin incision, to preserve tissue planes and ligate lymphatics with vessels for appropriate oncological control (see testicular biopsy).

Anatomical Points

Previous surgery may make orchidectomy more difficult; however, this is seldom a problem.

Table 5.6 Orchidectomy estimated frequency of complications, risks, and consequences

Complications, risks, and consequences	Estimated frequency
Most significant/serious complications	
Infection[a] overall	1–5 %
Subcutaneous	1–5 %
Systemic sepsis[a]	<0.1 %
Scrotal swelling[a]	50–80 %
Infertility	Definite
Rare significant/serious problems	
Bleeding/hematoma formation (scrotal)[a]	
Wound (immediate or delayed)	0.1–1 %
Wound breakdown/dehiscence	0.1–1 %
Seroma formation[a]	0.1–1 %
Wound sinus/suture granuloma	0.1–1 %
Chronic discharge	<0.1 %
Further surgery (delayed prostheses or hematoma drainage)	1–5 %
Implant problems (when used)[a] (dislodgment, infection, foreign body reactions, skin ulceration)	0.1–1 %
Less serious complications	
Residual pain/discomfort/tenderness	
Short term (<4 weeks)	50–80 %
Longer term (>12 weeks)	0.1–1 %
Loss of scrotal volume	>80 %
Sensory changes	<0.1 %
Psychological changes	50–80 %
Urinary retention/catheterization	0.1–1 %
Scarring/poor cosmesis	<0.1 %

[a]Dependent on underlying pathology, anatomy, surgical technique, and preferences

Perspective

See Table 5.6. Complications are generally minor; however, on occasions some may be more significant. These include bleeding, hematoma formation, infection, skin necrosis, wound dehiscence, cosmetic deformity, acute and chronic pain, and rarely recurrent hydrocele. Urinary retention is not uncommon and occasionally requires catheterization. Irreversible infertility is of course a consequence of this surgery.

Major Complications

Pain may be significant and may require support dressings and pain relief. Chronic pain occasionally occurs and is a major problem. **Bleeding** is rarely severe but can produce a large hematoma requiring surgical evacuation. **Infection** usually responds to local dressings and oral antibiotics. Infection may cause wound dehiscence, increase **scarring,** and create **poor cosmesis. Loss of scrotal volume** is usual, as expected, but this can be a significant problem especially for younger men and testicular implants may be desirable. When these are used, implant complications of infection, dislodgment, and skin ulceration are risks.

Consent and Risk Reduction

Main Points to Explain

- Discomfort/pain
- Infection
- Bleeding
- Delayed healing
- Wound dehiscence
- Infertility
- Cosmetic deformity
- Further surgery

Testicular Open Biopsy (Inguinal Approach)

Description

General anesthesia is almost always used; however, spinal anesthesia may be used. The aim is to deliver the testis from the scrotum into an inguinal incision to inspect the testis directly and perform a testicular biopsy. An inguinal incision is made on the side of the pathology approximately over the inguinal canal, and the external oblique fascia is opened. A wedge biopsy is taken of the testis in the relevant area of concern. The tunica albuginea is closed and the testis is returned to the scrotum, avoiding violation of the lymphatics draining either the testis or scrotum. The procedure is usually unilateral, unless biopsy of both sides is required. Orchidectomy can be performed for malignancy or suspected malignancy by this approach (see above).

Anatomical Points

The testis usually has a smooth outline and a firm consistency. Hard regions within the testis are abnormal. The epididymis is usually closely applied to the posterior aspect of the testis; however, it may be loose on a mesentery or lying anteriorly to the testis (in up to 5–10 % of cases). Epididymal cysts or hydroceles may obscure the testis, making surgery more difficult. Duplex ultrasound can be very reliable in determining the correct diagnosis.

Table 5.7 Testicular open biopsy (inguinal approach) estimated frequency of complications, risks, and consequences

Complications, risks, and consequences	Estimated frequency
Most significant/serious complications	
Infection[a] overall	1–5 %
Subcutaneous	1–5 %
Systemic sepsis[a]	<0.1 %
Bleeding/hematoma formation (scrotal)[a]	
Wound (immediate or delayed)	0.1–1 %
Scrotal swelling[a]	50–80 %
Rare significant/serious problems	
Wound breakdown/dehiscence	0.1–1 %
Seroma formation[a]	0.1–1 %
Sperm granuloma	0.1–1 %
Wound sinus/suture granuloma[a]	0.1–1 %
Further surgery (orchidectomy or hematoma drainage)[a]	1–5 %
Infertility[a]	<0.1 %
Chronic discharge[a]	<0.1 %
Less serious complications	
Residual pain/discomfort/tenderness	
Short term (<4 weeks)	50–80 %
Longer term (>12 weeks)	0.1–1 %
Sensory changes	<0.1 %
Psychological changes	50–80 %
Urinary retention/catheterization	0.1–1 %
Scarring/poor cosmesis	<0.1 %

[a]Dependent on underlying pathology, anatomy, surgical technique, and preferences

Perspective

See Table 5.7. Complications are generally minor; however, on occasions some may be more significant. These include bleeding, hematoma formation, infection, skin necrosis, wound dehiscence, cosmetic deformity, acute and chronic pain, and rarely ischemia of the testis. Urinary retention is not uncommon and occasionally requires catheterization. A potentially serious complication is infertility, due to excessive swelling of the testis after surgery producing increased intratesticular pressure and ischemia, where testicular atrophy may result. This may be significant if the other testis is also infertile or compromised and if fertility is desired.

Major Complications

Pain may be significant and may require support dressings and pain relief. Chronic pain occasionally occurs and is a major problem. **Bleeding** is rarely severe but can produce a large hematoma requiring surgical evacuation. **Infection** usually responds to local dressings and oral antibiotics. Infection may cause wound dehiscence, increase **scarring,** and create **poor cosmesis**. **Infertility** is a possible problem for men desiring childbearing ability.

Consent and Risk Reduction

Main Points to Explain

- Discomfort/pain
- Infection
- Bleeding
- Delayed healing
- Wound dehiscence
- Testicular atrophy
- Infertility
- Cosmetic deformity
- Further surgery

Vasectomy Surgery (Male Sterilization)

Description

General anesthesia is almost always used; however, local or occasionally spinal anesthesia may be used. The aim is to locate the vas deferens in each side and divide these to produce infertility. A separate transverse scrotal incision on each side, or a single midline incision, through the layers of the scrotum, is used, to expose both vasa. Several methods can be used, but a standard method is to excise a 1 cm section from each vas and then invert each cut end tying the end of the vas back on itself using nonabsorbable sutures. The cut ends are then inverted and physically separated. The scrotum is closed in layers.

Anatomical Points

The anatomy is usually fairly constant but can vary with previous surgery to the scrotum or testis. Duplication of the vas is extremely rare but can occur. Absence of the vas is also very rare. Physical examination preoperatively may define the anatomy reasonably accurately in most cases.

Perspective

See Table 5.8. Complications are generally minor; however, on occasions some may be more significant. These include bleeding, hematoma formation, infection, skin necrosis, wound dehiscence, cosmetic deformity, acute and chronic pain, and rarely

Table 5.8 Vasectomy surgery (male sterilization) estimated frequency of complications, risks, and consequences

Complications, risks, and consequences	Estimated frequency
Most significant/serious complications	
Infection[a] overall	1–5 %
Subcutaneous	1–5 %
Systemic sepsis[a]	<0.1 %
Scrotal swelling[a]	50–80 %
Infertility and irreversibility (essentially)[a]	Definite
Rare significant/serious problems	
Bleeding/hematoma formation (scrotal)[a]	
Wound (immediate or delayed)	0.1–1 %
Wound breakdown/dehiscence	0.1–1 %
Sperm granuloma	0.1–1 %
Wound sinus/suture granuloma	0.1–1 %
Persistent fertility/delayed infertility (< 12 weeks)[a]	0.1–1 %
Reanastomosis of vas deferens (spontaneous)[a]	<0.1 %
Duplicate vas deferens (v. rare)[a]	<0.1 %
Failure to locate the vasa[a]	0.1–1 %
Further surgery (hematoma drainage)[a]	0.1–1 %
Less serious complications	
Residual pain/discomfort/tenderness	
Short term (< 4 weeks)	50–80 %
Longer term (> 12 weeks)	0.1–1 %
Sensory changes	<0.1 %
Psychological changes	0.1–1 %
Chronic discharge	<0.1 %
Possible increased risk of arteriosclerosis/heart disease[b]	<0.1 %
Urinary retention/catheterization	0.1–1 %
Scarring/poor cosmesis	<0.1 %

[a]Dependent on underlying pathology, anatomy, surgical technique, and preferences
[b]Several previous studies indicated possible increased cardiovascular risk; however, large recent studies have essentially refuted this

rejoining of the vas. Urinary retention is not uncommon and occasionally requires catheterization. Tender sperm granuloma may cause chronic pain. Infertility is an intended consequence of the surgery, but the patient must understand that reversal may not be possible, and infertility may be permanent. Sperm samples need to be tested postoperatively, usually at 8 and 12 weeks, both requiring no motile sperm present to prove infertility has been established. There is a documented failure rate usually detected at the two sperm specimens, but even after these being negative.

Major Complications

Pain may be significant and may require support dressings and pain relief. Chronic pain occasionally occurs and is a major problem. **Bleeding** is rarely severe, but can produce a large hematoma requiring surgical evacuation. **Infection** usually responds to local dressings and oral antibiotics. Infection may cause wound dehiscence, increase **scarring,** and create **poor cosmesis. Failure to produce infertility** can occur from a variety of causes, including vas rejoining, failed vas ligation, poor contraception during the 12 weeks after vasectomy, duplicate vasa, and technical difficulties. **Spontaneous rejoining** of the vas is also possible, although uncommon, and usually occurs within 12 weeks, if it occurs. This is a rare cause of **persistent fertility**. Adequate ejaculations post-vasectomy must occur to clear the system of sperm, and **other contraception** is required until infertility is established. **Permanent infertility** is a possible problem for men desiring childbearing in the future, perhaps if circumstances were to change, which needs to be understood.

Consent and Risk Reduction

Main Points to Explain

- Discomfort/pain
- Infection
- Bleeding
- Wound dehiscence
- Permanent infertility
- Persistent fertility
- Contraception need
- Sperm tests
- Further surgery

Varicocele Repair (Inguinal Approach)

Description

General anesthesia is almost always used; however, spinal anesthesia may be used. The aim is to deliver the testis from the scrotum into an inguinal incision to inspect the testis and cord directly and repair the varicocele. Several techniques are used with the aim of ligation of the varicosities directly or the feeding vessels more proximally. The ligation may be performed in the scrotum, inguinal canal, or retroperitoneum. Laparoscopic approaches for the latter are relatively popular. For open surgery, an inguinal incision is made on the side of the pathology approximately over the inguinal canal and the external oblique fascia is opened. The procedure is usually unilateral, unless both sides are affected.

Anatomical Points

The testis is supplied principally by the testicular (L1 aorta) and cremasteric (inf. epigastric a.) arterial circulations, with a small contribution from the artery to the

Table 5.9 Varicocele repair estimated frequency of complications, risks, and consequences

Complications, risks, and consequences	Estimated frequency
Most significant/serious complications	
Infection[a] overall	1–5 %
Subcutaneous	1–5 %
Systemic sepsis[a]	<0.1 %
Scrotal swelling[a]	50–80 %
Further surgery (recurrent varicocele or hematoma drainage)[a]	1–5 %
Rare significant/serious problems	
Bleeding/hematoma formation (scrotal, inguinal, or retroperitoneal)[a]	
Wound (immediate or delayed)	0.1–1 %
Wound breakdown/dehiscence	0.1–1 %
Testicular atrophy[a]	0.1–1 %
Infertility[a]	<0.1 %
Wound sinus/suture granuloma[a]	0.1–1 %
Chronic discharge[a]	<0.1 %
Less serious complications	
Residual pain/discomfort/tenderness	
Short term (<4 weeks)	50–80 %
Longer term (>12 weeks)	0.1–1 %
Sensory changes	<0.1 %
Psychological changes	50–80 %
Urinary retention/catheterization	0.1–1 %
Scarring/poor cosmesis	<0.1 %

[a]Dependent on underlying pathology, anatomy, surgical technique, and preferences

vas (from sup. vesical a.). The pampiniform plexus of testicular veins is the main drainage and source of varicosities constituting a varicocele. Ligation of the testicular artery in the inguinal region (before or in the inguinal canal) can reduce the varicosities, with the remaining two circulations supplying the testis. Duplex ultrasound can be very reliable in determining anatomy and confirming the diagnosis. Varicoceles are more common on the left side due to a longer, more tortuous drainage route to the left renal vein. A true varicocele usually collapses on standing up. Obstruction of the left testicular veins at that level of the left renal vein, due to invasion of the renal vein by renal carcinoma, may prevent the collapse of the varicocele on standing (although a rare cause of varicocele).

Perspective

See Table 5.9. Complications are generally minor; however, on occasions some may be more significant. These include bleeding, hematoma formation, infection, skin necrosis, wound dehiscence, cosmetic deformity, acute and chronic pain, and rarely ischemia of the testis. Urinary retention is not uncommon and occasionally requires catheterization. A potentially serious complication is infertility, due to ischemia and atrophy of the testis after surgery. This may be significant if the other testis is also infertile and if fertility is desired. Laparoscopic approaches carry some additional risks of gas embolism, organ or vascular injury, and surgical emphysema, but these are usually rare.

Major Complications

Pain may be significant and may require support dressings and pain relief. Chronic pain occasionally occurs and is a major problem. **Bleeding** is rarely severe but can produce a large hematoma requiring surgical evacuation. **Infection** usually responds to local dressings and oral antibiotics. Infection may cause wound dehiscence, increase **scarring,** and create **poor cosmesis. Infertility** is a possible problem for men desiring childbearing ability.

Consent and Risk Reduction

Main Points to Explain

- Discomfort/pain
- Infection
- Bleeding
- Wound dehiscence
- Recurrent varicocele
- Testicular atrophy
- Possible infertility
- Further surgery

Further Reading, References, and Resources

General Urology

Smith and Tanagho's General Urology (Smith's General Urology) Series: Smith's General Urology 18th ed. McGraw-Hill Professional, 2012.

Circumcision

Bazmamoun H, Ghorbanpour M, Mousavi-Bahar SH. Lubrication of circumcision site for prevention of meatal stenosis in children younger than 2 years old. Urol J. 2008;5(4):233–6.
Bode CO, Ikhisemojie S, Ademuyiwa AO. Penile injuries from proximal migration of the plastibell circumcision ring. J Pediatr Urol. 2010;6(1):23–7.

Clemente CD. Anatomy – a regional atlas of the human body. 4th ed. Baltimore: Williams and Wilkins; 1997.

Heyns CF, Groeneveld AE, Sigarroa NB. Urologic complications of HIV and AIDS. Nat Clin Pract Urol. 2009;6(1):32–43. Review.

Jamieson GG. The anatomy of general surgical operations. 2nd ed. Edinburgh: Churchill Livingston; 2006.

Kim HH, Goldstein M. High complication rates challenge the implementation of male circumcision for HIV prevention in Africa. Nat Clin Pract Urol. 2009;6(2):64–5.

Perovic SV, Djinovic RP, Bumbasirevic MZ, Santucci RA, Djordjevic ML, Kourbatov D. Severe penile injuries: a problem of severity and reconstruction. BJU Int. 2009;104(5): 676–87.

Warner E, Strashin E. Benefits and risks of circumcision. Can Med Assoc J. 1981;125(9): 967–76–992.

Surgery for Meatal Stenosis

Clemente CD. Anatomy – a regional atlas of the human body. 4th ed. Baltimore: Williams and Wilkins; 1997.

Jamieson GG. The anatomy of general surgical operations. 2nd ed. Edinburgh: Churchill Livingston; 2006.

Bilateral Fixation of Testes/Exploration of the Testes

Clemente CD. Anatomy – a regional atlas of the human body. 4th ed. Baltimore: Williams and Wilkins; 1997.

Jamieson GG. The anatomy of general surgical operations. 2nd ed. Edinburgh: Churchill Livingston; 2006.

Hydrocele Repair

Clemente CD. Anatomy – a regional atlas of the human body. 4th ed. Baltimore: Williams and Wilkins; 1997.

Jamieson GG. The anatomy of general surgical operations. 2nd ed. Edinburgh: Churchill Livingston; 2006.

Epididymal Cyst Resection

Clemente CD. Anatomy – a regional atlas of the human body. 4th ed. Baltimore: Williams and Wilkins; 1997.

Jamieson GG. The anatomy of general surgical operations. 2nd ed. Edinburgh: Churchill Livingston; 2006.

Orchidectomy

Clemente CD. Anatomy – a regional atlas of the human body. 4th ed. Baltimore: Williams and Wilkins; 1997.
Jamieson GG. The anatomy of general surgical operations. 2nd ed. Edinburgh: Churchill Livingston; 2006.

Testicular Open Biopsy (Inguinal Approach)

Clemente CD. Anatomy – a regional atlas of the human body. 4th ed. Baltimore: Williams and Wilkins; 1997.
Jamieson GG. The anatomy of general surgical operations. 2nd ed. Edinburgh: Churchill Livingston; 2006.

Vasectomy Surgery (Male Sterilization)

Adams CE, Wald M. Risks and complications of vasectomy. Urol Clin North Am. 2009;36(3):331–6. Review.
Clemente CD. Anatomy – a regional atlas of the human body. 4th ed. Baltimore: Williams and Wilkins; 1997.
Jamieson GG. The anatomy of general surgical operations. 2nd ed. Edinburgh: Churchill Livingston; 2006.
Kaplan AI, Rappaport JA. The law and vasectomy. Urol Clin North Am. 2009;36(3):347–57.
Kotwal S, Sundaram SK, Rangaiah CS, Agrawal V, Browning AJ. Does the type of suture material used for ligation of the vas deferens affect vasectomy success? Eur J Contracept Reprod Health Care. 2008;13(1):25–30.
Lucon M, Lucon AM, Pasqualoto FF, Srougi M. Paternity after vasectomy with two previous semen analyses without spermatozoa. Sao Paulo Med J. 2007;125(2):122–3.
Practice Committee of American Society for Reproductive Medicine. Vasectomy reversal. Fertil Steril. 2008;90(5 Suppl):S78–82. Review.
Sokal DC, Labrecque M. Effectiveness of vasectomy techniques. Urol Clin North Am. 2009;36(3)):317–29. Review.
Trollip GS, Fisher M, Naidoo A, Theron PD, Heyns CF. Vasectomy under local anaesthesia performed free of charge as a family planning service: complications and results. S Afr Med J. 2009;99(4):238–42.
Trussell J, Lalla AM, Doan QV, Reyes E, Pinto L, Gricar J. Cost effectiveness of contraceptives in the United States. Contraception. 2009;79(1):5–14.

Varicocele repair

Clemente CD. Anatomy – a regional atlas of the human body. 4th ed. Baltimore: Williams and Wilkins; 1997.

Diamond DA, Xuewu J, Cilento Jr BG, Bauer SB, Peters CA, Borer JG, Mandell J, Cendron M, Rosoklija I, Zurakowski D, Retik AB. Varicocele surgery: a decade's experience at a children's hospital. BJU Int. 2009;104(2):246–9.

Jamieson GG. The anatomy of general surgical operations. 2nd ed. Edinburgh: Churchill Livingston; 2006.

Méndez-Gallart R, Bautista-Casasnovas A, Estevez-Martínez E, Varela-Cives R. Laparoscopic Palomo varicocele surgery: lessons learned after 10 years' follow up of 156 consecutive pediatric patients. J Pediatr Urol. 2009;5(2):126–31.

Mohammed A, Chinegwundoh F. Testicular varicocele: an overview. Urol Int. 2009;82(4):373–9. Review.

Salem HK, Mostafa T. Preserved testicular artery at varicocele repair. Andrologia. 2009;41(4):241–5.

Tong Q, Zheng L, Tang S, Du Z, Wu Z, Mei H, Ruan Q. Lymphatic sparing laparoscopic Palomo varicocelectomy for varicoceles in children: intermediate results. J Pediatr Surg. 2009;44(8):1509–13.

Index

Printed by Publishers' Graphics LLC
DBT140115.15.17.6